MW01631922

Sexual Health
Sexual Self

The importance
of sexual awareness
for relationships,
fertility, and family.

Dr. Habib Sadeghi

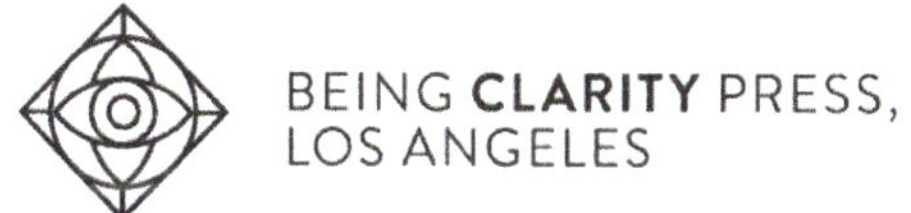

Sexual Health Sexual Self: The importance of sexual awareness for relationships, fertility, and family

The information provided in this book is not intended to be a substitute for medical advice, particularly with regard to any symptoms that may require diagnosis or medical attention. The reader should always consult his or her physician first regarding their current state of health and before making any changes to their lifestyle, healthcare practices, or plan of care.

Print ISBN: 978-1-966186-01-4 (paperback) 978-1-966186-02-1 (hardcover)
eBook ISBN: 978-1-966186-00-7

Published by Being Clarity Press
BeingClarity.com

To

Dr. Morton Herskowitz
for his invaluable mentorship in emotional armoring

and

Dr. Beverly Whipple
whose pioneering work in female sexuality helped me
understand the sexual response in women as no one else could

Other books by Dr. Habib Sadeghi

WITHIN: *a spiritual awakening to love and weight loss*

The Clarity Cleanse: *12 steps to finding renewed energy, spiritual fulfillment, and emotional healing*

MegaZEN: *Holistic health for the whole family*

CONTENTS

PREFACE

Sexual health is vital to overall health. From sleep, mood, and motivation to cardiovascular health and bone density, sexual health is an integral part of total wellness. At the same time, misperceptions about sex and our own sexuality can impact our bodies in ways that affect the delicate balance between emotional wellbeing and physical health.

I first became aware of this connection during my healing journey from testicular cancer while still in medical school. It was in my search for treatment alternatives that I began to understand the mind-body health connection and the impact childhood sexual abuse had on my perceptions of sex, my sexual self, and the part those emotional conflicts played in the manifestation of my illness.

Since then, I have seen this dynamic play out in many of my patients whose present physical disease is connected to an unresolved emotional issue from their past that is sustaining or preventing the condition from responding adequately to treatment. Like myself, these emotional challenges often involve conflicts related to sex and sexuality.

As a young physician of integrative medicine, it became clear to me that in order to give my patients the best chance at healing, their minds needed treatment as well as their bodies. That's what holistic healthcare is really all about and what it means to treat the "whole" patient.

As more of my patients revealed struggles with sexual issues regarding themselves or their intimate relationships, I became a certified sexuality counselor through the American Association of Sexuality Educators, Counselors, and Therapists (AASECT). In addition to a Master of Spiritual Psychology degree, extended mentorships with mental health experts like clinical sexologist Dr. Patti Britton and Dr. Jon Tabakin of The Psychoanalytic Center of California along with becoming an ordained minister, I've done my best to equip myself with the necessary tools to create holistic interventions for patients that bridge the gap between the physical healing they want and the emotional healing they need.

While I've shared some of those patient stories in this book, I also felt it was important to provide additional information to help readers better understand sex, sexuality, and intimate relationships. Many misperceptions about sex arise from our fear of talking about it, especially to our children, but fear breeds ignorance and the consequences that come from bad choices.

With that in mind, I've done my best to offer inspiration for healing while also including guidance on improving communication and bonding in intimate relationships, how to talk to children about sex without instilling shame or judgment, protecting children from internet pornography and its negative impact on relationships, how to disagree with your partner without devolving into drama, and the best way to end a relationship without bitterness and emotional baggage. All these things can help prevent the kinds of misunderstandings and emotional scars people often acquire from sexual issues early or later in life that eventually impact their health.

At the same time, you'll find information on addressing important sexual health issues such as fertility struggles, maintaining healthy hormone levels while aging for men and women, the problems with prostate and breast cancer screening, why so many women can't reach orgasm, how much sex is okay during pregnancy, and other topics. It's my hope that through sharing what I've learned and a deeper understanding of the synergy between sexual, emotional, and total health that you'll enjoy a greater level of wellness and a richer life experience in your relationship.

INTRODUCTION

According to the World Economic Forum, the yearly global cost for treatment of chronic diseases will soon reach $47 trillion.[1] In the U.S., costs related to chronic diseases already consume 90% of the $4.5 trillion spent on healthcare annually.

When it comes to diseases like cancer, neurological disorders, auto-immune conditions and others, it's clear the healthcare industry is woefully inadequate at eradicating the diseases it has become so effective at diagnosing over the last 70 years. This is due in part to the idea on which so much of modern medicine is founded. The human body is seen as a collection of organs and systems that perform separate functions. Only in the most rudimentary of ways are these ever considered related one to another with virtually no attention given to the body as an integrated whole.

This idea has led to the increasing specialization of healthcare which further fragments the body into ever-smaller components. The current approach healthcare moves treatment further away from the idea that it's the interrelation between the parts of the body as a whole that results in wellness.

Given the continued rise in chronic disease costs and the fact that modern medicine has little to offer but symptom management, perhaps it's time we take an approach that focuses on harnessing the body's ability to eradicate disease by restoring its *own* equilibrium. For such an approach to gain widespread approval, it would be necessary for it to be tested in the same manner applied to all large research studies each of which requires empirical evidence. Given the deep financial alliances between pharmaceutical companies, the major universities, and accredited journals that publish the findings of such studies, how likely is this? Do these conflicts of interest that prevent studies of large-scale mind-body medicine from ever happening or being published in most mainstream medical journals mean those treatments don't work?

There is a reason that mind-body medicine is the fastest growing field in healthcare. The new understanding of brain chemistry is a remarkable achievement in that we no longer regard the physics of the chemical body as all that makes for wellness, so much so that it has bred whole new categories of treatment—psychology and psychiatry. The mind's ability to influence the body is now a standard way of looking at biological processes and wholeness or whole-body health.

As I ponder the current challenges of healthcare, I think back to how some of the most radical changes in medicine came about. One of the most notable discoveries ever made came from Hungarian physician Ignaz Philipp Semmelweis. Today he is known as the Savior of Mothers. In the 1800s, puerperal fever, bacterial infections of the reproductive tract after child birth also known as childbed fever, was rampant and claimed the lives of many new mothers. Semmelweis showed how death rates could be reduced to less than 1% if doctors simply washed their hands between treating different patients.

Because his observations went against established medical opinions of the time his ideas were rejected. While Semmelweis had no formally researched explanation for why his conclusions were correct, all the anecdotal evidence he brought forward from his personal practice with new mothers proved he was right. Even so, without the support of the medical establishment his recommendations were ridiculed. Some doctors even took offense at the suggestion that they were somehow "unclean" and should wash their hands between delivering babies. The debate became a controversy and at age 47 Semmelweis was committed to an asylum where, after being beaten by guards, he died two weeks later. It took years for Louis Pasteur to introduce the world to the existence of bacteria and vindicate Semmelweis' recommendations about physician cleanliness forever.

Given this example and many others I would argue that anecdotal evidence is a legitimate part of the initial research process and should never be dismissed out of hand. Just because there isn't $10 million available to conduct a five-year, double-blind study on 2,000 patients doesn't mean a treatment doesn't work. On the contrary, there is an incredible amount of empirical evidence that some of the therapies I will present in this book are changing lives. You need no convincing if you are a patient whose chronic health problem of 10 years or more was resolved in a matter of days or weeks by these so-called novel approaches.

Like most doctors, my medical education and initial career focused only on the body. Over a period of time, it became obvious that my patients' state of mind also played a part in their health. Earning my master's degree in spiritual psychology with its emphasis on consciousness took me into a deeper exploration of how the mind interacts with the body to impact health.[2] Much of this has to do with how each of us, to varying degrees, carries unresolved emotional issues from our past and how we physically resist or "armor" ourselves against feeling or fully processing them.[3]

Over time, it's the long-term psychological stress from these unresolved emotional issues and the biological and/or chemical changes they trigger in the body that eventually transform the mental upset or dis-*ease* into a physical disease. This is usually the case when a patient doesn't respond to traditional treatment. In those situations, I've found there is a long-term emotional imbalance of some kind helping to sustain the physical imbalance in the body. In order for the body to respond properly to treatment, the unresolved emotional issue must be diagnosed and treated, as well.

One example is David, a 69-year-old CEO of an international pharmaceutical corporation, who came to me at the behest of a friend. Our initial conversations didn't go well. He wasn't open to anything I had to share and flatly stated at our first meeting that he had only made an appointment with me as a favor to his friend whom I had previously treated. "This is rubbish," he said as he hung up on me after calling to tell me he was quitting therapy.

David had stage IV prostate cancer. It had metastasized to the bone and was unresponsive to treatment, including radiation and chemotherapy. When his friend heard about how he had ended our conversation, she insisted he call me back and continue our work together. "If there is any chance left for you to heal," she said, "this is it." With all other options exhausted, what did he have to lose?

We began our discussions by talking about emotional trauma. "I haven't had any trauma," he flatly told me. I explained how trauma is relative to each person, encouraging him to share his story over the coming weeks. As he did so, I saw how he had experienced more than his share of trauma.

David was born in France and from his earliest years he felt estranged from his mother. She clearly showed preference for his brother for whom all her time and affection were reserved while David's accomplishments went unnoticed. One day, in front his brother and a group of friends, his mother said of her eldest son, "I know he's going to be a great artist someday, but David? I have no idea where he'll end up."

It wasn't long before he was assigned to a Canadian nanny who whisked him off to Canada to finish the rest of his growing up. Eventually, he moved to Los Angeles where he met and married his wife, Karen. At that point, his life was looking up.

In addition to fathering a beautiful daughter, David became CEO of one of the largest pharmaceutical corporations in the world. Despite his success, his mother still refused to acknowledge his accomplishments or have any contact with his daughter. "She's all the way over there in the United States," his mother said. "She'll never know me anyway."

Years later after arriving back in Los Angeles after a business trip, David was surprised to find his father-in-law and a family friend waiting to pick him up at the airport instead of his regularly scheduled driver. On the ride home, he discovered that while he was away Karen had died from an undiagnosed heart condition.

David shut down. Unable to properly grieve, he packed up Karen's belongings and locked them in the attic. Every video, photograph, or greeting card that bore her image or handwriting was piled into a suitcase and left to linger in the darkness with his memories of her.

Four months later, David was invited to a dinner party where he met Cheryl. Soon after meeting, they married.

When David came to see me, he was living in Europe and had been battling cancer for years. He was also displeased with his daughter, Grace. Now in her 30s, she was lazy and overweight, according to him. David was concerned she wasn't dating or making any effort to move her life forward.

I explained to David how, in the case of men, the pain of rejection and abandonment by the women they love is most often deposited in the sexual or urogenital organs of the body. Being rejected by his mother disrupted his root chakra, the energy center in the body that provides us with our sense of safety and security in the world. This energy center surrounds the perineum and base of the spine, including the area of the prostate. Unresolved issues of rejection and abandonment by the opposite sex in men will lead to energetic disturbances in these areas and eventually disease.

From my observations, feelings buried alive never die. David thought he had escaped the pain of his past when what he had really done was stuff it down inside himself just as he had done with the suitcase in the attic that held every memory of Karen.

In order to heal, I told him that he must begin to properly grieve first for the loss of Karen, then for a mother's love that would never come. Even though David had liquidated all of Karen's belongings years before moving to Europe, he still had the suitcase with all of her videos, cards, and photos. After so many years, he needed to take a trip back to the attic and allow himself the dignity of his own emotional process. Once he released the emotional charge from Karen's death, I felt quite sure his body would respond in kind.

In an incredible act of bravery, David allowed himself to view the old home movies of Karen and read her beautiful words to him. Not long after, he called to tell me that for the first time ever his cancer was responding to treatment. Even his relationship with Grace was benefitting from his emotional and energetic shift. They were getting along better, and she was making plans for her future and dating again.

It didn't happen overnight, but David's regular physicians in Europe have officially declared him to be in remission. He continues to do work on honoring his emotional process in all areas of his life.

As David's case demonstrates, a mind-body approach is crucial when it comes to freeing ourselves from the many ways in which our bodies engage in armoring as a result of emotional trauma. With the consent of several of my patients whose stories I will relate, this book will explore numerous ways in which emotional armoring affects our health.

Today more doctors and patients are joining a growing consensus that lasting health comes from the synchronization of mind and body as a single unit not from further hyper-specialization that continually breaks the body down into an ever-increasing number of otherwise autonomous parts and then treats those parts in isolation. When something is synchronized, it means that its separate parts work together as a whole to achieve a common purpose. If even a single element is out of place, the outcome could be completely different.

To see the power of synchronization, look at a clock. The intricate gears and weights work together in absolute precision in order to track the time within a fraction of a second. Equally, all parts of an Indy 500 race car, including the driver, interact tens of thousands of times to execute a superior performance that gets across the finish line first.

We've all seen movies where someone flips a hidden switch that triggers lots of gears and gizmos that interact in just the right way to open a secret door. Regardless of the disease one may be dealing with the goal is always the same, to *re-synchronize* the system.

In a sense, there aren't lots of cures for lots of different diseases but one cure that touches them all. When I and other physicians like me speak of health, what we really mean is a human body where the various parts are working in a coordinated fashion for the wellness of the whole.

Coordinating thousands of different organs, tissues, fluids, hormones, and cells to work together in harmony might seem like an impossible task, but it's not a matter of working with all these elements separately. That really would be impossible. To deal with a system as complex as the human body, it's best to take a holistic top-down approach. To the degree that we affect the elements at the top of such a system, all the parts and processes below that level are also modified and in turn function in a more cohesive way because they're all interconnected.

This is where sex enters the picture. In a synchronized environment that functions as originally intended, disease cannot exist. One of the hormones released from the pituitary gland as a result of sexual activity is oxytocin. Oxytocin is showing promise not just in helping to bring the body's biological systems back into a coordinated state but also as a powerful agent in fighting existing disease. Tumor cells have receptor sites for oxytocin, and *in vitro* lab studies have shown oxytocin to inhibit abnormal cells in the outer layer of breast tissue and uterus, as well as in bone.[4] *In vivo* tests showed oxytocin continued to inhibit proliferation of breast cancer in mice and rats.[5]

While oxytocin's healing properties show promise with some types of cancer, results also revealed that its presence may work to assist the proliferation of other types such as prostate[6] and those involving the endothelium or primary cell layer of certain body cavities.[7] In the absence of these cancers, however, oxytocin's ability to synchronize all body systems via the brain's central nerve zero (CN0) is immeasurable. In Chapter 5, we'll look at how it's able to do this.

Much of the healing benefit we gain from the presence of oxytocin arises out of the moments of mutual bonding that author Barbara Fredrickson calls "positivity resonance." In her book, *Love 2.0,* she states that during these moments of intimacy the brain syncs up with another person in a shared empathy that she refers to as "brain coupling" or two people having a singular experience. We listen more during the interaction and even anticipate the other person's needs and intentions. This state is important for health because it facilitates deep connection and improves the synchronicity of our relationships.[8]

"There is no illness of the body apart from the mind," said Socrates more than 2,400 years ago. The term psychosomatic comes from the ancient Greek language where *psycho* means *mind* and *soma* means *body*. The ancient Greek healers knew that all illness was a psychosomatic, mind-body event that required treatment on both fronts. Sadly, today we use the term to imply that an illness is "all in the head" or imaginary which isn't the case.

The vast majority of diseases is psychosomatic and has its origins in the mind which generates our thoughts. These thoughts give rise to our emotions which resonate at the cellular level. The quality, consistency, and intensity of those emotions generate biological changes that produce the physical printout we call the body and its current state of health.

With this understanding, it becomes clear that in order to heal a physical disturbance or disease of the body we must first heal the related emotional disease present in the mind. This is why *psycho* comes before *somatic*. All disease and healing begin in the mind and end in the body. It's for this reason that we speak of illness as a dis-*ease*, pointing to something going awry within our psyche first.

This was the case with Kelly, a film producer. For as long as she could remember, she was always on her own. Her father, a Moroccan diplomat, was constantly traveling while her American socialite mother had an equally full schedule that kept her away from home. When her parents did manage to spend time at home, it was usually filled with fighting.

Eventually, the extended separations and disagreements brought her parents' marriage to the breaking point. One day while her father was on a business trip, Kelly's mother told her they were taking a vacation. It was only after they left Morocco and settled in the U.S.

that Kelly learned they were there to stay.

When Kelly's father discovered their whereabouts, he made his way to the U.S. to meet with her mother who wanted a divorce. Kelly's father pleaded with his wife to stay in the marriage. He told her that he wanted to have another child but had no interest in doing so with another woman.

In Kelly's words, her parents made a "business decision." Her mother offered to have another child but on the condition that they not move back to Morocco. She wanted to live in France. Kelly's father agreed to the deal.

Shortly after the family set up their home in France, Kelly's mother told her of her intention to have another baby. Upon hearing the news, Kelly protested, "Are you crazy? You can't have another child. Dad's constantly traveling and you're never around. This is going to be a disaster. You know who's going to end up raising this child? Me!"

That's exactly what happened. Kelly's parents had a son, but their respective schedules barely missed a beat in terms of their international and social obligations. Kelly's childhood was bluntly interrupted by having to raise her brother and step into the shoes of a mother who wasn't there.

Thirty-three years later, Kelly was sitting in my office fighting thyroid cancer. When she shared her story with me I asked her, "Can you spit?"

Instead of looking at me like I'd lost my mind, Kelly responded, "Oh my God. How did you know? My dad used to try and teach me how to spit, but I could never do it."

I explained to Kelly that in my experience of working with patients with thyroid cancer this one question easily determines if their problem originates in the psyche. Those who cannot spit have a strong psychic element involved in their condition. On an unconscious level, the inability to spit represents not being able to separate that which we want to keep from that which we want to expel.

In Kelly's case, her protest against her parents having another baby fell on deaf ears and she felt impotent and ineffectual. She had gone through life not speaking up for herself. She couldn't separate the good from a situation while rejecting the bad and moving on. She took all the responsibility upon herself and kept it inside, especially in relationships.

I shared with her that all thyroid conditions reflect an energy imbalance in the throat chakra. Not being able to spit means not being able to express ourselves or our needs. Kelly found out early that her needs didn't matter and stopped expressing them. Even decades later when her wedding planner spent three times her budget, she said nothing.

As an adult, Kelly had no relationship with her mother. I explained that when motherhood was forced on her, her superego moved into the mother role, consuming her and not allowing her true self to develop. In doing so, it caused her to merge energetically and unconsciously with the internal object of her greatest pain, her mother. The result was that Kelly had no idea who she really was.

Stuck in the mother role decades after her brother had grown up, at work she was the one everyone came to for advice, dumping all their problems on her. She was the one they turned to for comfort, caring, and direction. The constant counseling of others was burdensome, but Kelly couldn't speak up and set boundaries.

I found out how deeply Kelly was stuck in a motherhood mentality when she told me that her husband was impotent. She knew it when they married. They had never had intercourse. This was quite telling because Kelly felt impotent her entire life and could never assert her opinion when it mattered.

Kelly's husband's behavior was adolescent much of the time. She told me several stories including one where her husband was baking a pie. When he opened the oven door to check on it, he tilted the tin too far and spilled some of the filling onto the burner below. He immediately reacted with such hysterics that he burst into tears.

"Kelly, do you realize that you're not a wife in this relationship?" I asked her. "You're the mother. You married a man-child, a baby."

Even her previous relationships included men who were not assertive, needed coddling, or were looking for a mother figure. She had spent her life finding herself inexplicably drawn to people who needed saving, protection, and guidance.

The key for Kelly was to learn to pay attention to how she was relating to herself internally in each situation and to express those needs in the moment. By stating what we need, we create experiences that help us discover who we are and what we're about. Kelly needed to make herself the focus of her own life. The child she had to save was the one inside of her.

After much internal work, Kelly was able to set up boundaries in her professional and private life. She also had a heart-to-heart discussion with her husband stating that, as his wife, she deserved the pleasure of having intercourse with him and that it was his responsibility to seek out the necessary treatment to make that happen.

In psychosomatic illness, consciousness precedes form. All Kelly's work helped her step out of the mother mind and into her own personhood. When this shift happened in her consciousness, her body shifted as well.

By speaking up for herself in many areas of her life, Kelly is now able to spit for the first time. She has learned how to speak her mind and expel what she doesn't need from her life. She has done much work nurturing her inner child and continues in the process of forgiving her mother. Her reward was to be declared cancer-free.

The traditional approach to medicine has convinced most people that the body is just a lump of flesh which is why we feel it's the doctor's job to make us well. We are completely oblivious to the many ways the mind is the map or operator's manual from which the body functions. We fail to recognize that finding the mental or emotional root of an illness, the psychic portion of the healing process, comes before or together with addressing the secondary bodily effects of those psychic patterns. This gives us as patients a responsibility for our healing that goes far beyond just taking our medications as directed. It's emotional or mental work that enables the prescriptions, supplements, treatments, and surgery to do their part in the healing process.

Healing is a partnership. As the patient commits to doing the necessary psychic work of emotional healing, the doctor gets busy working on the somatic aspects of restoring the body. The extent of the physical healing that takes place is contingent upon the level of emotional healing that occurs. This means the emotional aspect of the healing process is by far the most important part of any treatment protocol.

It's for this reason that some patients heal spontaneously without any significant physical treatment whereas others see their diseases return despite extensive medical interventions. *Healing is an emotional transformation rather than a physical manipulation.* This is good news because it means the power to get well has been placed firmly in the hands of the patient. In fact, that's where it's always been.

Health or disease is predominantly the product of our thoughts and emotions, and no one gets to think our thoughts but ourselves. There is a great deal of power and freedom in that realization. When an illness strikes, it's easy to panic and frantically look outside ourselves for a solution, for the next doctor, hospital, or treatment that we believe is the Holy Grail of our healing. Instead, illness is an invitation to quiet the mind and look inward. The task is to examine our hearts and souls for unresolved emotional issues from our past that may be generating unhealthy conscious or unconscious thoughts and emotions that have been harming our bodies long before physical symptoms appeared.

Illness is a call to emotional action not a summons to attack a physical disease. It asks us to become aware of an unconscious emotional thought pattern that's limiting our lives in a significant way. This means that while illness may look like our enemy it's actually our ally in healing at a deeper level. Enough time has passed that the body has chosen the quickest and most obvious way to show a person that something beyond the physical needs healing. When this issue is recognized, resolved, and finally released, the result is a better quality of life that's free from the interference of our old beliefs and their associated limitations.

It can be frightening being diagnosed with a serious illness. As patients, the temptation is to focus all our efforts and consciousness on fighting its physical manifestation. My suggestion is to leave that to the doctor. *Your work is internal.* As patients shift their focus to healing emotionally, physical healing will follow as a natural byproduct.

Everyone needs support on their healing journey in service of their return to health. As we are about to find out, in no area of our lives is this more important than our sexuality. Along the way, we'll explore how to strengthen the bonds in our intimate relationships, how to put sex in a positive context for our children, and how to make the best choices when it comes to our sexual health. All these things are necessary if we wish for a balanced and fulfilling life because sexual health is a vital part of total health.

Chapter 1

Sex as a Meditation

Sexual energy is spiritual energy

Sex. Few words command so much attention. Simply mention the word and images of everything that's innocent to indulgent flash across people's minds. Sex is provocative and personal. Everyone seems to have an opinion on it including when to have it, how to have it, with whom, and for what reason.

One question many people can't seem to answer is whether sexual energy is spiritual. In this book, we're going to examine how sexual energy does indeed function as spiritual energy. In order to understand sexual energy in a spiritual context, it's necessary to temporarily suspend all the opinions we have about it. Spiritual energy is pure consciousness. It's the great oneness out of which everything is created. Without it, nothing would exist.

Spiritual energy can take any form depending on how it's channeled through you. If you're angry, joyful, or sad, it becomes emotional energy. When you explain to someone how to use a computer program, it's mental energy. During a rigorous workout it becomes physical energy. All energy is spiritual in the ultimate sense because everything comes from spirit. Sexual energy is the form spiritual energy takes on when something new is to be created. This can—although not always—involve having children.

Artists of all kinds, particularly actors, singers, and dancers often describe their performances as sexual in nature. This doesn't mean in an erotic sense necessarily but as having the same freedom and power to command someone's attention as happens in a sexual encounter. This is no surprise since the sacral chakra, the energy center which controls all creativity, is located between the naval and pubic bone. It also happens to govern the reproductive organs. As such, creativity is sexual energy which is spiritual energy because it's the nature of spirit to create.

Sexual energy is why we exist, to continuously create new things and experiences to learn from. It's through this continuous process of creating, learning, and then creating something else from what we've learned that our consciousness evolves to higher levels. Since none of us would be here without sex, we are all equally spiritual *and* sexual beings.

Passion & Purpose

Tantra is the Hindu-Buddhist process of liberating or separating consciousness from physical matter. It's a practice by which we transcend the physical limits of the body and experience our true nature which is eternal consciousness through a sexual meditation. According to Swami Satyananda, tantra comes from the Sanskrit words *tanoti* (expands) and *trayoti* (liberates). Knowing this, how then does sex expand and liberate us?

The level of spiritual satisfaction we currently enjoy in our sex lives is largely dependent on our past experiences, our judgments about sex, the kind of sex we're having, and why we're having it. Some tantra philosophies have defined four different types of sex each with its own specific purpose. These include procreation, recreation, restoration, and transformation.

Most of western culture is stuck in the first two categories. We have sex to create children for our families which is a noble act. After all, the human species does have to go on. Having sex strictly for the second reason or physical pleasure is great but in itself is the lowest application of this powerful energy.

While sex is certainly a means of procreation, this shouldn't be its end. Neither should sex be performed as a marital "duty" which does a great spiritual disservice to both people involved. The ultimate goal of sex is to provide the path to a higher purpose.

It's understandable why we in the western world would choose to have sex for practical and physical purposes without much spiritual depth. Nonstop exposure to hyper-sexualized images in advertising, television, film, and pornography have left us struggling through superficial and transient relationships, disconnected from our creative passions and lacking spiritual power. To this we can add the stifling, shame-based religious dogma that often makes sex taboo to talk about and one of life's baser elements.

Deeper Connection

Have you ever looked into the eyes of the person with whom you were having sex? What did you see there? I'm talking about looking at them protractedly as you orgasm, peering into their soul during that brief but intense moment of oneness and connection.

Did you see a person whose eyes have a light in them, a light that lets you know they're fully present with you in a way that moves and uplifts your spirit? Deadened eyes can't look for long at a person whose eyes are bright and alive. It's been said that no characteristic of the human body reveals so much as do the eyes. What do you convey through your own eyes during this most intimate of human acts?

The eyes project inner power and the contents of the soul which is why we often prefer to avoid direct eye contact with other people. Getting locked in a gaze with someone can quickly leave a person feeling vulnerable and emotionally exposed with no way to hide their inner feelings and insecurities. Standing in an elevator demonstrates very well why we avoid eye contact most of the time, especially with strangers, to the point of totally ignoring someone else's presence.

Just as the eyes are the primary vehicle of flirtatiousness, they are the portal through which you and your partner allow as much or as little sexual energy to flow between you. As psychiatrist Morton Herskowitz concluded after years of seeing patients, "Everyone who fantasizes when he makes love is escaping from his mate with his eyes. Full, clear eye contact is necessary for total involvement."

The eyes have been described as the mirror of the soul, and not just the eyes, but the expressions so many of us wear. Walk down an average street in a large city. What do you see on the faces of the people walking toward you?

We all have our moments of happiness but nevertheless ours is not what I would describe as a deliriously happy world. As I walk down the streets of any major city, I see more furrowed brows than smiling cheeks. Even when I encounter a smile, it often seems forced instead of emanating from the heart. I see expressions that tell of pain and strain more than of joy and exhilaration. I see eyes that are more filled with anxiety than peace.

It's been said that some of the characteristics the eyes convey are sneaky, tricky, guilty, self-effacing, excited, mean, sad, bitter, cynical, scared, lively, ardent, hopeful, trusting, and joyful. To read eyes deeply is to be exposed to the pain, anger, and dismay of the human species. People suppress such pain and sorrow in their lives that it has become second nature. It's gotten to the point where we can't feel or even recognize our own pain any more than anyone else's. It's like we've made an unconscious agreement with one another saying, "I'll pretend you're happy if you pretend I'm happy."

Emotional Armoring

It isn't only the eyes that are affected by how we feel but the breath. People seem barely alive as they go about their daily duties. Look at the chest of the average individual. It's tight and sunken forward with shallow breathing. It's as if the central role of breathing is to act as an energy inhibitor whose task is to put a damper on deep emotions. It's not by chance that the heart and emotions of love are linked. We have learned not to *feel.*

Everything from a person's facial expression to their body carriage and how they walk across a room is an indicator of the way their body has armored itself against feeling emotions. Even those who think of themselves as "spiritual" people and in tune with their subconscious patterns may well have forgotten what it means to feel. This is often the case with my patients such as Anne who, through no fault of her own, had shut down her ability to feel until disease arrived.

"I don't understand it," said Anne when I first met her. "I eat all organic and have practiced transcendental meditation for over 20 years. How does someone like me get cancer?"

Anne felt betrayed by her body. How could someone who did all the right things the media experts said were necessary to avoid cancer end up with breast cancer at that time in her life?

The first point I shared with Anne was that while diet and lifestyle are an important part of healing, they were only a part of the process. Based on my personal experience with cancer many years ago and hundreds of patients since then, diet and lifestyle are about 30% of the healing equation. The real healing shift comes from the other 70% of the process which involves finding the emotional component that's supporting the *dis*-ease and doing the necessary psycho-spiritual work to release it.

This is why, despite eating right, exercising, and meditating, cancer will always return after surgery, not because the doctors didn't "get it all out," but because the emotional undercurrent that was feeding the entire process at the cellular level was never addressed.

One thing I noticed about Anne's overall personality that I thought might be a clue to an underlying unresolved emotional issue was how she felt about men. Although she was married, Anne had an extremely negative attitude toward men so much so that some might have classified her as a man-hater.

Through our work together, I discovered a childhood trauma where Anne's mother, who was being beaten by her husband, escaped into the bathroom and locked the door. Anne, who was already in the bathroom, suddenly found herself trapped with her mother while her father raged on the other side of the door. She was 11 at the time.

Anne said it was this experience that led her to resent and mistrust men. Eventually, she married but by her own admission Anne had only had sex with her husband a handful of times.

Two months after having her daughter, Anne's husband returned from an out-of-town bachelor party acting disrespectfully. The situation escalated until her husband finally admitted he had a one-night fling with another woman. For Anne, this confirmed all of her negative perceptions about men. Instead of leaving her husband immediately, she chose to stay with him because she wanted a second child. The baby came, but nothing else changed. A couple of years later, Anne was diagnosed with breast cancer.

Sitting in my office, Anne said she couldn't stand her husband and reiterated that they had only been sexual a handful of times since they had married. Her husband was now drinking and overweight.

I shared with Anne that unresolved emotional issues regarding the opposite sex, whether it be a parent or partner, often manifest disease somewhere in our sexual organs. If cancer had an emotional calling card, it was *resentment*. Anne's years of resentment toward her father then her husband and men in general was the cancer that was eating away at her. Resentment is one of the most common emotional precursors to cancer.

Anne eventually made the decision to have a mastectomy but without radiation or chemotherapy. I stressed to her that unless she did the proper work and dissolved her emotional buildup of resentment there was no guarantee her cancer would remain in remission. To her credit she got to work, particularly with creating authentic communication with her husband and her father with whom she hadn't spoken since college.

Anne recently celebrated her 17th wedding anniversary. She enjoys a renewed and fulfilling relationship with her husband who has lost weight and is getting his life back on track. They even have sex three times a week! She's had her father over for dinner several times, and they too have come to understand each other better.

Worthy to Receive

Imagine how different the quality of our lives and relationships might be today if we understood that sexual activity, either alone or with a partner, can be the gateway to a greater version of ourselves. To share such a union with someone is the closest we can come in this existence to oneness with the divine source from which we all originate.

As distorted as many of the ways in which we share sexual energy have become, it's also through sex that we can experience healing. Even so, such healing doesn't come from the promiscuous "free love" kind of casual sex that was first introduced to people in the 1960s and now in the Internet Age rebranded as "hookup" culture.

For the creative nature of sexual energy to be physically and emotionally healing, all that's required is to be able to receive the love contained within a meaningful sexual encounter. To receive love, we must know that we are worthy of it.

Have you noticed the hard and coarse manner in which many people deal with each other today? It goes well beyond common rudeness and seems as if they're saying to each other, "You got a problem with me? You don't like it? Well, fuck you!" The same callous and selfish nature in which those people live their daily lives they also take into their sex lives and intimate relationships. The hardness or crudeness with which they make love is telling, usually seeing their partner as nothing more than a vehicle for their physical pleasure and a way to "get off." Subconscious pain is frequently associated with "hard fucking" and often manifests itself in degrading or humiliating sex acts and even rape fantasies. The anger and contempt underlying this pain often speak to how so many people screw one another both inside and outside the bedroom these days.

Slow touch is as much a key aspect of making love as is sustained eye contact. The kind of frantic sex glamorized in films that has both partners ripping each other's clothes off is supposedly a sign of passion, but it's really a reaction driven by the anxiety of *not* wanting to feel authentic emotion either from themselves or the other person. This kind of disconnected, autopilot consciousness is indicative of how we engage with most other aspects of life, as well. We have become so habitually entrained to fending off our anxiety in this manner that we don't realize how often we're "checking out" of our lives even as we live them.

Neutralizing Negative Emotions

In preagricultural times, people were generally less anxious than we are today. How do we know this? There are societies on earth far from modern civilization that live much the same way they did thousands of years ago. This includes the stone-age Tasaday of the Philippines or even the premodern Eskimos among others. Because they're less emotionally armored in their approach to each other, they transmit much through touch.

The sexual urge generates the momentum of life's productive energy so much so that it could be said sexual health is a barometer of human health and wellbeing. It's only when we are sexually free—which doesn't mean we take a hedonistic approach to sex—that our full potential to experience, produce, and create is realized.

When we are sexually free, we are alive in the most primal sense. Because we have greater access to and consciousness of our emotions as human beings, we experience the whole spectrum of our senses more fully in every aspect of our lives, including the times of sorrow and pain.

The effect of fully experiencing our emotions can be dramatic. In the case of rage, the difference with feeling intense anger as a fully conscious individual is that as it arises in the mind, it's allowed to build to a natural climax and then pass through and out of the body, leaving no negative energetic residue. The negative charge is fully felt, processed, and neutralized without allowing it to stagnate in the mind and thus become embedded or armored in any part of the body to eventually create disease. The result is the ability to fully manage one's emotions without being unconsciously driven by them, in this case rage, and to no longer be an angry person.

When it comes to good health, the ability to fully process our feelings in this way is essential for all emotions. Consider grief as an example. If we are experiencing grief either through the death of a loved or some other reason that removes that person from our lives, we grieve on multiple levels. Our grief arises not only from the togetherness we will no longer share with that person but also the circumstances surrounding the separation, our feelings of powerlessness to change it, and the void we feel from their physical absence. All these variations of grief must be recognized and released to fully process such a painful experience.

Feeling all our emotions in their completeness is how we live a conscious life and maintain present moment awareness no matter what may be happening to us. The point of consciously feeling isn't to feel better, it's to feel *everything*.

Wonder as a Way of Being

When nature stirs within us a sense of wonder and creates the feeling of happiness, the fleeting sensory experience is awakening something deeper within ourselves—something that, though we may be unaware of it, has been there all the time. That something is pure joy, the contentment and peace that are intrinsic to our spiritual nature and humanity. In other words, beauty and majesty don't cause this joy; they evoke it. It's already within us waiting to be awakened.

There is wonder to be had in the ordinary, everyday things of life if we allow it to emerge. Wonder isn't just a response to something wonderful; it's actually a way of being. It happens when we stop taking things for granted and pay closer attention to the smaller aspects of life. If we allow ourselves to be amazed by how dewdrops cling to a spider's web in perfect symmetrical rows or the earthy smell of fall leaves as they crunch under our feet it can awaken an innocence in us that fills every day with all kinds of new discoveries. Wonder as an approach to daily life is what grounds us in present moment awareness and prevents us from getting stuck in regret and resentment of the past or worry about the future.

It's not just sexually but in every aspect of their lives that most people can find themselves in an emotionally armored state, rigidly retaining feelings they're either afraid or unable to fully experience. This means, on the whole, that the world is also in an armored state with the pent-up anger, resentment, frustration, pain, loss, and insecurity of hundreds of millions of people constantly being misdirected at each other and their environment every day. How else can we explain why humans seem so bent on poisoning nature and their own food with toxic chemicals or the way they prey on each other with things like "cancel culture", physical violence, frivolous lawsuits, and of course, war. How can we evoke a sense of wonder within ourselves when we're entrenched in such a morass of negative energy? The conflict and misery we see in the world every day only mirrors what is within us. *As above, so below; As within, so without.*

The Superficial Self

With so many people repressing their true emotions, it's no surprise that the feelings they do allow themselves to express are full of fake sentiment. So often a cashier at the grocery store or gas station takes your money and responds blandly, "Have a nice day." Do you ever get the feeling that they *really* want you to have a nice day? Probably not. It's so common for people to thoughtlessly ask someone else, "How are you?" without *really* caring about how the other person is actually doing emotionally or physically. Living among so many emotionally armored people means living in a world of feigned politeness and detached civility that leaves us stuck in an emotionally shallow existence starving for real connection.

On the rare occasion that connection does happen, it's unmistakable. It's like a little jolt of electricity or taking a drink of water after being desperately thirsty for a long period of time. That feeling of connection, being recognized, and relief is the feeling of your soul being fed. We feel this instant joy when we interact with small children and our pets because they have no emotional filters so the connection is always real. At the same time, trying to fool them with fake sentiment never works because they haven't learned to emotionally compartmentalize and are always clued into the energy of their relationships. They can always tell what we're feeling regardless of what we say.

The superficial self we present to the world that people confuse with who we really are is a learned self. It's an artificial persona we gradually put on like a mask as we grew up. We adopted it as we were told by adults not to speak unless spoken to so, we learned to bottle up our emotions along with what we wanted to say. At the same time, we learned a kind of superficial "niceness" because we wanted to be liked and receive acceptance.

Even if we're aware that this inauthentic, socially acceptable persona isn't who we really are, who we *think* we are still isn't our true nature either. T.S. Eliot tells us in his poem Four Quartets that only in ending the façade can we find the beginning of who we really are.

Into another intensity
For a further union, a deeper communion
Through the dark cold and the empty desolation,
The wave cry, the wind cry, the vast waters
Of the petrel and the porpoise. In my end is my beginning.

Life challenges us to rethink who we are. Everything that happens to us, disastrous as some of it may seem, forces us to reevaluate and ultimately reinvent who we are as a result of those experiences. Are we really the person we present to the world or even to ourselves?

Early Recognition

An infant forms its sense of who it is through the way it attaches to its caregivers. When a child cries or screams and the parents are upset because the situation is inconvenient—or later in life, the growing child dares to voice opposition—it learns through its caregivers' various reactions that to express itself is unwelcome.

When a child's gaze earns no reaction from its indifferent or busy parents, it learns to look less intently and disconnect from others and the world around it. The eyes lose their sparkle as the child's inquisitiveness and interest in life fade. How else do we explain why so many children who, as toddlers, were interested in everything transform into disaffected teens who want to drop out of life? Not acknowledging a child's presence and need to bond or express itself stunts its social, inquisitive, and creative energies.

Answering a child's question with the dismissive catchall response "Because I said so" with no explanation is to disregard the child's humanity not to mention throw away an opportunity for a teachable moment. As a result, the child grows up feeling that it's not just his voice that doesn't matter but by extension *he* doesn't matter. This is the core of poor self-esteem. Alternately, the child's subconscious reaction could swing in the opposite direction, leading it to adopt an inflated sense of self and a big ego. Add to this the shame-based effects of religious dogmas as well as the intense pressure to conform that comes from the educational and social systems, and it's plain to see why so many children emotionally armor themselves against a world that rejected their willingness to connect when it was offered.

As Karol Truman said, "Feelings buried alive never die." The unresolved emotions we consciously or subconsciously armor ourselves against don't simply go away after the experiences that gave rise to them end. The residual negative energy from those repressed feelings has lasting effects which, sooner or later, will manifest in our bodies or behavior.

Let's consider the shame and fear-based beliefs much of religion has associated with masturbation for boys. A child who is deprived of naturally and innocently exploring his own body will do it anyway but in a manner that feels sneaky and where sex must be "taken" when it can be had. This can lead to a young man objectifying sex and his sexual partner as something that can be possessed for his own pleasure. Suppressing sexual desire in this way often leads to outbursts of sexual behavior that are hurtful and unhealthy for both partners.

In contrast, a girl who grows up with shame surrounding masturbation and sexuality learns that sex is a duty, a service she provides to her husband for mostly his—as opposed to her—pleasure. As a result, she grows into a young woman finding herself in relationships where her intimate needs aren't met and abuse can happen. The natural instinct to love tenderly and passionately has been undermined by crude impulses. Sadly, this dysfunctional sexual dynamic can seem normal in a society that has replaced true intimacy with superficial fetishes and fantasies.

When feelings that are perfectly natural have been stunted from their full expression, they become a part of our minds that we call the unconscious. This is a complex collection of unexpressed emotions and repressed memories, mostly outside the realm of our immediate awareness, that exerts a powerful influence over our everyday actions. Until our eyes are opened to these hidden influences, we have no sense of how they affect our behavior and biology. To heal from illness, it's essential to work through unconscious emotional patterns that can manifest as or support diseases.

An Unwelcome Admission

Stephen, a partner in an investment firm, was suffering from three autoimmune conditions in which his body was creating antibodies that were attacking his own tissue. Vitiligo was causing him to lose the pigment in his skin, creating blotches all over his body as the melanocytes in his skin cells continued to die. Psoriatic arthritis left him in so much pain that among his arsenal of prescriptions was

Methotrexate, a medication normally given to cancer patients. At the same time, Hashimoto's thyroiditis was attacking his thyroid, creating severe hormonal disruption throughout his entire body.

I asked him to close his eyes and think of an experience in his life that he would consider traumatic. I had barely finished my request when he replied, "I'm already there." During his wedding reception, his father approached him, threw his arm around him, and said, "Stephen, I wish you and your new wife all the happiness in the world, certainly more than your mother and I ever had. Of course, that's why I've been cheating on her for years."

I asked Stephen how long ago his symptoms began. He told me two to three months after his son was born, he started to have arthritis pain. The other conditions followed soon after. When Stephen as the son became a father, he subconsciously turned the years of anger he held toward his dad for cheating on his mom against himself.

We sat in silence for a moment, but I could see he was already lost in another memory. As respectfully as I could, I asked him, "I was wondering what the possibility might be that you had a similar experience as your father?"

Stephen's eyes widened and began welling up with tears as he answered, "I don't know what you're talking about."

I simply observed, "It seems to me you're becoming emotional."

Stephen admitted, "If I understand what you're asking me, it's very traumatic."

Keeping the momentum going, I responded, "What do you think it is that I'm asking you?"

He said, "You're asking me if I've cheated on my wife."

I replied, "That's exactly what I'm asking you. Has that been your experience?"

Stephen said yes, going on to share how he had been having an affair for quite some time and had fallen deeply in love. Just before he was getting ready to tell his wife he wanted a divorce, she told him she was pregnant. He chose to keep his secret and stay in the marriage for the sake of the child.

The birth of his son was the trigger that turned Stephen's subconscious loathing for his father against himself because of his own infidelity. He had truly become his father. He felt he deserved to be punished which is why his body began attacking itself through three different autoimmune diseases.

Stephen was also filled with doubt, particularly about the kind of father he would be. If he chose to get divorced, he doubted having the respect of a son who only saw his father part-time and who would eventually discover the offense he committed against their family. If he didn't get divorced, would the love he had finally found go away?

I began working with Stephen to release the anger he felt toward his father and himself. We also spent much time learning how to live with uncertainty and the peace that comes from not needing to answer all the what ifs of his life.

In just a couple of weeks, Stephen's joint pain had improved so much that he was off the Methotrexate and his thyroid levels started normalizing. The erosion in his joints stopped as they began building new structure. In many ancient healing philosophies, the bones symbolize integrity because they give the body its structure. When Stephen reclaimed his own integrity, his bones responded.

The red blood cells of patients with cancer and autoimmune diseases burst after just two to three minutes in a saline solution because the cells have so little integrity. Stephen's were the same. After working together for several weeks, his red blood cells remained intact in saline for nearly 18 minutes, almost the average for healthy cells which is 20 minutes.

As Stephen continued to heal, he chose to make the decision that was most authentic for him which was to follow his heart and be with his new love. This change generated additional improvements for him as he continues to move toward a full recovery.

Living from Spirit

The unconscious mind starts to become cluttered with unresolved emotions early in life from the resistance we feel when asked to do things that aren't true to who we really are. It can start with something small like being required to kiss Aunt Martha every time she visited and, of course, she liked to kiss on the lips. Ick. Later, it can come from your parents requiring you to play a sport in school but you hated sports, or not being able to pursue something you actually loved like music. All these experiences leave their emotional signatures large and small on the subconscious over time, but we've buried most of them in the rush to get on with life.

We all understand how babies are innocent and yet, most of us eventually come to see ourselves as flawed either from the faults of others projected onto us as children or through religious dogma that says we are somehow broken or "sinful" from the beginning. This is especially the case when it comes to sex. Adam and Eve in the garden had their eyes opened and, suddenly realizing they were naked, became ashamed and embarrassed of their nakedness. What is it about nakedness that causes all the problems?

It's during sex that we have the opportunity to be seen, felt, touched, and heard at the deepest level. It's where we are the most exposed. Yet it's during sex that we hide the most. The honesty and vulnerability can be so intense that we resist full emotional engagement and hide not only from our partners but from ourselves, as well.

If we are ever to access our deepest self, we must work through all the ways our unconscious blocks us off from that core identity. It's from there that our deepest feelings arise along with our true purpose, free from the labels, limitations, and expectations of others about who and what we should be. In that state, we're vibrant, generous, socially conscious, and emotionally available in relationships. It's to be alive in every moment, consciously connecting with others and the world around us in a genuine way.

When our outward expression finally reflects our inner self, there is no division between the divine and everyday life; living becomes a spiritual experience. With subconscious false beliefs and limitations out of the way, we're naturally drawn to the people and opportunities that can help us create a more authentic life. This includes things like a job that's truly fulfilling and not just a paycheck, opportunities to express our creativity and empowerment, and relationships that are lasting and supportive.

When we live from our inner being, spirit permeates all we do. To be in touch with the realm of spirit is to be attuned to the wonder of reality. Rather than imagining spirituality as an ethereal state separate from our physical existence, we see and experience the divine as interwoven with the here-and-now. To live from spirit as our actualized selves is to be part of an all-embracing reality that immerses us in wonder as a way of being.

When you stare at a sunset do you really think the rush of wonder and peace you feel is supposed to be a momentary experience? It isn't. It's the beauty of your true self resonating with the beauty of nature because it comes from the same divine source. The spirit immersed in wonder is an intensely personal and yet universal experience.

As wonder becomes central to our existence, the artificial barriers we've put up between ourselves and the rest of the world begin to fade away. In the process, we see our interconnectedness with everyone and everything around us. Not only does this realization eliminate the desire to pursue superficial happiness through materialism but we shed our ego to exist in the world in a more mutually supportive and cohesive way.

A sexual relationship between two partners who know how and choose to share their core selves with each other can become a unifying expression of the divine source from which they both have their origin. In oneness, there is wholeness, equilibrium, and healing. When sex is understood in such a way, it has a healing effect unlike any other. If we thought of sex in this context, I'm certain most of us would have very different values with regard to sex and sexuality. We would have no difficulty in rejecting the sexual shame and fear taught to us by others. We'd also make better choices when it comes to with whom we share our sexuality.

Making these kinds of choices requires a deep sense of respect for ourselves and others. When we teach our children that sexual energy isn't an external aphrodisiac but part of who they *are*, self-respect and better choices happen naturally.

In life, we are all on a journey of first discovering the true self and then transcending it into oneness. Wonder is the experience of knowing ourselves as part of that all-encompassing mystery. As a sense of wonder invades our being through meaningful sex, we find ourselves identified with the whole pulsating energy of existence.

Giving over our body and spirit together to a lover in the act of conscious sexual union, we are more fully ourselves than at any other time. Our consciousness, spilling over its imaginary walls into all the universe that encompasses our partner, stretches ecstatically toward the mystery of being in which we and the universe are grounded.

Chapter 2

Why We Resist Passion

Orgasm isn't everything

The oldest bottle of wine in existence dates from AD 325, and a keg of wine from 1472 is still drinkable. In 2010, a group of Finnish divers found 168 bottles of 200-year-old champagne in a shipwreck. When one of the bottles popped open on its own, the divers dared a taste. Not only was the wine better than they expected, even a sommelier said it had a freshness and wasn't debilitated in any way.

Wine has long had a sacred significance. In addition to being a beverage, it was also used for medical purposes until the dawn of modern medicine. A jar containing wine and other medicines was found in the tomb of one of the first pharaohs of Egypt, Scorpion I. When civilization began to emerge from barbarism, wine played a part in extending Greek cultural practices across the world into countries such as France, Italy, and Russia.

Given its perceived ability to combat disease, soothe emotional pain, and make celebrations merrier, there is little wonder why wine became a metaphor for what it means to be human. What isn't often realized is that wine's potency to create these effects comes from grapes being *crushed.*

Grapes have within them just enough sugar to feed the yeast living on their skins that do the work of fermentation. The sugar is only released to the degree that the grapes are crushed. More crushing means more sugar is released and thus a greater level of fermentation. This is what gives wine its potency. As long as the yeast and sugar continue to interact, a good wine will mature over time.

Think about your life as a fermentation metaphor. How many

times have you found yourself feeling crushed by the circumstances of life, thinking that everything was ruined only to come through the experience wiser, stronger, or even grateful?

Much like wine matures, so do human beings. In our case, fermentation of the soul happens to us in our relationships, especially our more intimate ones. When the breakdown starts to happen and the condition of the relationship enters the acidic stage, many abandon the process. We trade the eventual sweetness of an exquisite cabernet sauvignon for the taste of vinegar. If we can recognize that the acid in our relationships has a higher purpose than just the sourness we experience at a particular moment, we can work with it and allow the breakdown to transform those partnerships into something sweeter.

Me vs. We

Whenever a couple is having trouble in their relationship, I invariably find that it revolves around the clash between the desire to be an individual and the desire to be together. It's in this struggle that we learn how to be an individual without losing ourselves in the relationship. It's the process through which our true self ripens.

If we are to become the best version of ourselves through learning, growth, and overcoming subconscious limitations, then it can only be accomplished in our relationships as we act as student *and* teacher simultaneously with our partners. This kind of deep healing and transformation can't happen in isolation. Human connection is the womb from which the fully developed self is born. It's in this psycho-spiritual evolutionary process that our full humanity is realized.

When I speak of *crushing*, the kind of breaking down to which I'm referring includes all the irritations, frustrations, resentments, and upsets that challenge us in relationships. These are the acidic experiences that drive the entire evolutionary adventure. The person we find ourselves to be today is the result of a continuous breaking down that led to a building up at a higher level, one that heralds our *becoming*.

This process exists between two people even as they share intimate moments. Imagine what it would be like if you and your partner came together with the intention of experiencing divine union in a love that's deeper than the physical, a love that enables you to become more than you have so far thought yourselves to be.

Deemphasizing Orgasm

In ordinary sex, orgasm is always the final target. It's the big prize, the reward for a job well done. We've glorified it so much that it has now become the holy grail of sexual union. It's *why* we do it, to release. Even people who consider themselves spiritual make the mistake of thinking that orgasm is the height of the sexual experience. It isn't.

The good news is that the spiritual elements within our sexual energy can be activated at any time. For a start, it means letting go of the standard routine of "first I do this, then you do that." The spiritual approach to sex produces a much more intuitive, evenly paced, and free-flowing experience.

This doesn't mean that every sexual encounter has to include two hours of foreplay. It means that the intent to achieve a deeper connection is present before each encounter and is the main goal. Orgasm and even intercourse are no longer the centerpiece of the experience. If they happen, that's great, but they are never the predetermined destination of a sexual encounter.

The spiritual path is all about the journey and not the destination. With this intention, each sexual encounter becomes more spiritually and emotionally satisfying while at the same time more erotic because it's completely unpredictable. This is the path to a truly transformative and physically transcendent experience.

A spiritual approach to sex provides us with the opportunity to heal in a multitude of ways. I'm sure there have been times after intercourse when you experienced the need for an emotional release. Perhaps you wanted to cry, laugh, or even scream. These emotions are triggers for subconscious memories or traumas that need to be released.

When these kinds of healing opportunities come into play, it's a great blessing but only if we are with a partner who can offer spiritual support. Only a loving environment where we feel safe enables us to experience our feelings to the fullest and bask in the restorative power of sexual energy.

At times, emotional triggers will arise long before orgasm. The person experiencing the emotional upheaval tends to stifle their feelings out of fear of breaking the sexual momentum and upsetting their partner. We can't be open to release and restoration through sexual energy if we're racing toward orgasm. When we take the emphasis off orgasm, we can be open to wherever each sexual encounter takes us.

Healing Potential

Consider for a moment the idea that you attracted, just like a magnet but through spiritual energy, your present partner into your life. Since opposites attract, you drew someone to you whose disposition, habits, and behaviors run counter to yours in certain ways. Simultaneously, your partner drew you to themselves by the same energetic process. While some of your characteristics may seem to clash with each other, the differences actually help balance your relationship and provide opportunities to learn and grow as individuals and a couple. Maybe you tend to have a short temper but your partner is more level-headed. Perhaps you're better in a crisis while your partner is prone to worry. Every irritation or conflict we have with our partners is an opportunity to look inward and ask ourselves, "What is it *within me* that attracted this situation into my life or what unresolved emotional issue in *my heart* could the situation be triggering that needs healed?"

Spiritually speaking, you attracted a partner who has the potential to help balance and heal your old emotional injuries if you're willing to look inwardly instead of attacking outwardly in those challenging moments. Growing up emotionally is a process, and some of our issues in need of healing may even have been mirrored back to us by our parents.

To see how this works, stick out your right hand with the fingers apart then weave the fingers of your left hand into those spaces. When you're old enough to be drawn to a partner, you'll draw someone to you not merely by physical attraction or sexual energy but also by spiritual energy, ultimately coupling with someone who has the necessary energetic makeup that can help reveal and/or fill those unconscious empty spaces in your heart.

These hidden hurts and undeveloped aspects of our identity form the basis of our unconscious mind. Because they're unconscious and, for the most part, we're unaware of them, we're attracted to partners who will draw them out of us where we can see and heal them. On the plus side, new positive qualities like courage, compassion, or determination are also brought forward as we face these challenges. They become our tools in the healing process.

The psycho-spiritual balancing act that happens between us and our partners feels good initially when the relationship is exciting and new. As we get to know our partners and the nuances of our personalities come into conflict, it becomes more challenging. When our unresolved emotional issues begin to get triggered on a regular basis, the situation feels threatening and all we want to do is bail out on the relationship. If we can resist this urge to blame and escape while looking inward for the unresolved emotional issue the outer drama is triggering, growth and healing can begin.

In some situations, it becomes clear that while we take this journey of self-discovery and healing, we cannot remain partners with the other person and need to move on. Handling the separation with a higher level of consciousness that doesn't allow the breakup to descend into drama is not only essential for your continued emotional healing and growth in the process, but it will protect your family and finances from going to ruin in a nasty divorce. We'll look at how this can be accomplished in a later chapter.

A Passionate Need

As old unconscious hurts are brought forward and healing happens, it allows the partners in a relationship to connect on a deeper level and engage in passionate loving. This doesn't mean wild, unrestrained sex but a more intense sense of oneness. Feeling this natural progression build toward a deeper connection, many people experience their emotional vulnerability for the first time and short circuit the process. They pull away and distance themselves emotionally while their bodies go through the motions of the physical act because being fully engaged in giving all of themselves to another person is just too scary. It would be easy to assume everyone wants to be loved passionately, but that's really not the case or so it seems. In fact, so many people subconsciously resist the invitation to love and be loved passionately that it could be argued they really *don't* want to feel loved, heard, and supported. Even so, at their core, they know passionate love is what their soul needs.

Gail Godwin's novel *Evensong* is the story of how a female minister named Margaret plans to marry a male chaplain, Adrian. When Margaret was a child, she was afraid that a witch would grab her and put her in a closet. Now, as she approaches marriage, a girlfriend reminds her of the scary witch story from her childhood and suggests that Adrian is a grownup version of the witch.

When we first meet our partners, they're perfect in our eyes. They're Prince or Princess Charming and can do no wrong. Actually, it isn't fair to hold our partners to such standards of perfection and to put them on a pedestal, but that's the effect of the euphoria of first falling in love. It's why they say love is both magical *and* blind.

Unfortunately, it doesn't take long before your partner's hidden pain and humanness come to the surface as the "witch" appears. "My God," you ask yourself, "did I pick the wrong person?" You thought you had picked the perfect partner and now this person looks like the embodiment of your worst nightmare.

When the witch appears in your relationship, it feels like everything is going wrong. This is because it's not the prince or princess who is going to enable you to fulfill your dreams of happiness and healing; *it's the witch.* She's showing you the aspects of your true self that haven't yet developed. You'll either continue to face her and work through the process to improve yourself and your relationship or she'll reveal to you why you attracted such an unhealthy relationship in the first place and give you the courage to moved forward out of it.

Early in Godwin's novel there is a description of a character called Madelyn of whom it's said that she "could see around to the backsides of the stage sets people presented as their lives." I believe that's what relationships are meant to do, enable us to see around to the backsides of the stage sets we present as our lives to other people. Of course, the fictional play we present to others along with the character we pretend to be in it isn't who we *really* are. It's in relationships of every kind, though especially the romantic ones, that we truly find out who we are. It's through our interactions with each other that we learn about ourselves and begin to see the incredible person hidden behind the masks we wear.

Writing to Margaret who has suggested that marrying him might limit him, Adrian asks, "Why would you be limiting me? Why shouldn't our having each other make more of us both?" This is the question we all need to answer with our partners. Why aren't we continuously working to improve ourselves individually and together in our intimate relationships to expand the experience for both people?

We might liken this to how every person produces an energetic "vibration" that draws them together with their appropriate partners. Psychologically, we can say the unconscious mind creates our life experiences based on the deepest beliefs we hold about ourselves and the world around us. Through our thoughts, feelings, and actions it causes us to seek out opportunities and situations that create similar experiences for us based on those unconscious beliefs.

Ease & Errors

The unconscious mind functions automatically and is always seeking to maintain order in our personal world *as we see it*. It doesn't matter whether the perceptions we hold about ourselves, another person, or a situation are true. The unconscious is completely neutral and non-judgmental. It behaves this way for two reasons.

The first is to make our lives easier so we don't have to think about a lot of things. When you were first learning how to tie your shoes, you had to consciously focus on every step of the process. If you knelt down to tie your shoe right now, your hands would fly through every one of the steps without even having to think about them. This is great when it comes to helping us effortlessly navigate the many mundane aspects of life. Things become habit.

The unconscious also seeks to make greater order out of our personal world by leading us into situations that are guaranteed to confirm our existing beliefs, right or wrong, and challenge us to confront those ideas in order to learn and grow. Virtually all of our beliefs about ourselves and the world around us were neurologically wired by approximately the age of eight. This creates a big problem for most of us who grew up in a less than ideal environment. We drew all sorts of unconscious conclusions about ourselves based on our interactions with the world around us, thereby creating unconscious behavioral programs that run our lives today.

If you pay attention, you'll notice that humans tend to act in *unconscious* but *predictable* ways when we find ourselves in certain situations that are similar to a previous experience. Automatic actions directed by the unconscious mind might be convenient for tying our shoes but it becomes damaging if we integrated the assumption as a child that we didn't deserve to be loved. As a result, such a false belief will unconsciously drive a person to seek out situations and relationships where love is withheld and they are treated poorly no matter how badly love is wanted.

Perhaps you are familiar with the axiom, *As above, so below.* It tells us that whatever thoughts are allowed to dominate the mind they will eventually affect the body. In the same way we could easily say, *As within, so without.* Our outer life circumstances always reflect our inner beliefs about ourselves and the world. At first glance this might seem depressing, as if we are doomed to be automatons, regulated by unconscious beliefs we have no access to and that limit our lives.

As we uncover the unconscious beliefs that have been holding us back, creating the same kinds of problems in our relationships or causing us to attract the same type of person becomes less likely. Living in a more conscious way, we can create new beliefs that drive different choices that better serve us.

Understanding Projections

An important part of this change process is understanding how projections work in relationships. While our unconscious thoughts aren't immediately accessible to us, they make themselves known in our reactions to the situations in our lives. There's an old saying, "You spot it, you got it." It means that we can't get offended by any characteristic within another person unless we also have a corresponding element of it in ourselves.

Because the unconscious mind isn't accessible to us directly, it has a way of getting our attention by causing us to project our beliefs outward onto other people. This is what is meant by the term projection. By becoming aware of the ways in which we project our fears, faults, and insecurities onto other people, we discover those issues are actually true of ourselves and need healing.

I'm sure you've had a coworker say or do something that irritated you for some reason. While their behavior got on your nerves, why didn't it affect every person in the office the same way? It's because they didn't have a similar belief in their unconscious that resonated with that person's behavior. What *you* took to heart, *they* could ignore.

A movie projector can only reveal the images on a filmstrip by projecting them onto an external surface. In the same way, your unconscious mind uses other people and situations as a screen so you can become aware of the limiting beliefs you hold about yourself. This enables you to neutralize them and move toward a better life.

Take a look at the judgments, irritations, and outrage you express toward other people. Instead of ranting at someone you feel doesn't respect you, consider that your unconscious mind is acting like Gail Godwin's witch. The witch has created an experience of someone disrespecting you to try and wake you up to the fact that you unconsciously don't respect yourself. Why else would you continually put yourself in the company of people who treat you badly?

If this doesn't work to get your attention, your body may try next. As a physician, I can't tell you how many people come into my office complaining about things like neck stiffness, indigestion, and acid reflux. If no physical cause can be found, I always ask them about the quality of their current relationship. I'm not surprised when they respond, "My husband is *such a pain in the neck*." Another patient says, "Things have gotten so bad, *I can't stomach it anymore*."

When we fail to understand the messages we project onto others, we continually inject ourselves with negative emotional energy that harms our health. That's when the body starts talking to us, and there's no better way to get our attention than with pain.

Feeling is Frequency

When it comes right down to it, there is no "out there" in life. Every person or situation we experience, positive or negative, is reflecting back to us some aspect of ourselves. If it pleases us, that's great. If not, then we must begin the work of discovering the false belief that supports it and change it. It's the only way any significant change can happen in life. This is why trying to change someone else is always an exercise in futility.

Scientifically speaking, a new belief brings with it a new feeling, and a change in feeling is a change in energy or frequency. This means that we'll begin attracting to ourselves people and situations that match our new energy and validate the supportive belief we now hold about ourselves.

We may also be surprised how the existing people in our lives start showing up differently without our even having to ask them to change in any way. If they don't respond positively to our new energy, our frequencies will be incompatible and they will fade out of our lives. If nothing else, life is a continuous series of self-referral experiences designed to increase our individual awareness so that we can create better lives for ourselves.

Regardless of whether we experience something as good or bad, our only response to it should be directed inward. We should ask ourselves, "What does this have to say about me? Why did I make the choices that got me into this situation? What did I do or what do I think that led me to attract this same type of person into my life?" While a situation from our past or even distant past may not seem to be associated with our current troubles, much of the time it is.

Laura came to me because she had gained a significant amount of weight over the previous two years and it was impeding her job performance as a corrections officer in the men's wing of the county jail. After diets, exercise regimens, and other interventions didn't work, she suspected a hormonal problem might be the cause.

When her hormone panel came back normal, I learned that she hadn't been in a relationship for several years prior to taking on her new job. When I asked her how she felt about this, she said she was fine with being alone. Eventually, she would reveal that she had been sexually assaulted in the years leading up to her job at the corrections center but that, emotionally speaking, she had "worked through all of that."

I politely suggested that might not be the case. Her inexplicable weight gain could be a subconscious protection mechanism to keep men, who she now felt were dangerous, away by making herself unattractive to them. When we subconsciously feel we are in danger and need to protect ourselves, the body will find a way to armor itself against the perceived threat. Laura was armoring herself with fat.

I presented her with results from a heavy metals toxicity test she had taken during her first visit. Her levels of mercury, aluminum, and cadmium were through the roof. As such, she was also *literally* armoring herself against men with metals.

Even the job she had taken as a corrections officer in a men's jail mirrored her subconscious need to be in a position of authority over men. Her work involved seeing how the bad guys were being punished. With access to guns and the men securely behind bars, she gained an additional sense of safety.

Over the course of the next 18 months, I put her on a detox protocol for the heavy metals and worked with her to identify and express her repressed emotions. By the end of that time, she had returned to her normal weight.

I tell all patients and clients I mentor, "How you relate to an issue *is* the issue, not the external details of the situation." To look outside ourselves for an answer is to stay mired in unconsciousness, recreating the same negative experiences again and again.

Doing the Work

The following seven-step process is a tool I developed to help clients work through issue resolution within their relationships. This is a self-reflective exercise designed for one person. For the purposes of this exercise, we'll use the example of a wife who feels that her husband fails to appreciate everything she does for the family.

Step 1
Recognition

It's important to recognize that a problem exists in your relationship. This might seem simple, but too many times one or both partners move through their lives in avoidance or denial that anything is wrong just to "keep the peace."

Eventually, the pent-up pressure becomes too great and explodes into a volatile situation that could have been avoided. It's also important to admit that this problem is drawing your attention to a deeper issue within yourself that's limiting your life in some way. It isn't necessary to identify what that issue is at the moment.

This is also where you get in touch with the anger, sadness, rejection, jealousy, or other emotions you're feeling. Perhaps you consider yourself "spiritual." Perhaps you believe that spiritual people shouldn't experience negative emotions. In truth, the *only* negative emotion is the one that's *repressed.*

Find a place that's private where you can give yourself enough time to fully release what you're feeling. If you want to yell and scream at a photograph of your partner, you can do that. If you prefer to beat your mattress with a tennis racquet pretending it's your partner's head, that works too. It's essential to fully realize and release what you're feeling. You don't want to stay this upset long-term, but it's important to face up to how you really feel.

This action recognizes your emotions as valid and helps you move into the rest of the exercise with a more neutral, less emotionally-charged frame of mind.

Step 2
Commitment

Set a clear, positive intention to resolve this situation within yourself and make a commitment to do the necessary work to see its outcome manifested in your life. In the case of our example, it might sound something like the following:

> *My intention is to heal the source of the hurt and anger inside of me that I feel when my husband ignores all that I do for the family. I will embrace what I learn about myself from this situation to bring peace and clarity to my life.*

It's best to write your intention down. Since it has been proven that goals are more often accomplished when they are written down, writing has a powerful effect on the subconscious. This also provides a way of making your commitment to yourself more real by bringing it out of the mind and into the physical world. Read your intention out loud often as a means of recommitting yourself to the work.

Step 3
Ownership

Here is where the blame game ends and you accept 100% responsibility for creating the situation as you currently experience it in your life. This doesn't mean you are responsible for your partner's actions or that anyone is condoning what he or she is doing. Even so, you are entirely responsible for the emotions you feel and how you are experiencing the situation through the filter of your unconscious perceptions.

The situation is no one's fault; there is no right or wrong here. It's just an experience generated from your subconscious mind that's providing you with the opportunity to heal an old emotional wound, reclaim a disowned aspect of yourself, and live more fully as the person you really are. To do this, you must acknowledge that the situation is acting as a trigger for a deeper hurt inside of you. This hurt is calling out for healing through the use of a projection from your subconscious mind.

Claiming 100% responsibility for all the conscious and unconscious thoughts and actions that created the current problem provides you with all the power needed to change the situation. This is because once you discover the unconscious limitation your projection is trying to bring to your attention, you can consciously choose your response the next time your partner exhibits the behavior in question.

The minute you make someone else responsible for any part of your life or your feelings, you have entered a *victim mode* and made yourself their *prisoner*. Since you tell yourself you can't be happy until they change, you've left them in charge of your happiness. This is the fast track to a lifetime of powerlessness and misery.

Changing people is an inside job. The only person you'll ever be able to change is yourself but it requires taking full ownership for every thought, belief, action, and choice you've ever made that has brought you to this moment. When you realize that it's only you who can make choices in your life, you will witness your anger transform itself into empowerment.

Take some time to write out a statement similar to the example below, inserting your own details. Sit with it for a moment, then read it aloud a few times. If you have any resistance to the statement, you'll feel it in your body. In that case, you may need to release more anger as stated in step one. In the example of a wife who feels her husband doesn't appreciate all she does for the family she might write the following:

> *My feelings are my responsibility. No one can make me feel anything. I recognize that my feelings arise from the judgments I place on a person or situation based on the subconscious perceptions I have about myself. When my husband doesn't take notice of all that I do for the family, the upset I experience is a trigger for a deeper hurt that is trying to get my attention. I blame no one for this situation, including myself, and claim 100% responsibility for every thought, belief, emotion, and action that has manifested it in my life. I understand the real purpose of this situation is to realize and release a limiting belief I have about myself that's been keeping me from being more of who I really am. I welcome this change and move forward in non-judgment for my highest good.*

Step 4
Inner Treatment

In this step, it's necessary to go inward and establish a dialogue with your authentic self whether you call it your higher self, higher power, spiritual essence, or something else. This is the state of mind many people enter during meditation. This is the highest part of your consciousness that holds all the answers you are seeking.

Prior to this exercise, take a moment and write down all the emotions you feel regarding your partner and the situation. Don't focus on the details of who did what but how those things *made you feel* and the judgments you placed on the other person.

With eyes closed, take a few deep cleansing breaths. Sit for a few moments in silence and let the thoughts of the day fade out of your mind. In a calm and respectful way, ask either aloud or mentally to be able to connect with your authentic self. Wait for a few moments. There may be a slight deepening of your meditation, a sensation of warmth, or a sense of calm that washes over you.

After another moment, focus on the emotion from your list that affects you the most. Try to embody it as much as possible, allowing it to flow through you. Ask your authentic self to show you the moment in your life when this feeling had the most significant influence on you. Sit with the sensation and see what comes forward. Move through the emotions on your list and allow your authentic self to reveal the hurt from the past that's being triggered by your present situation.

In our example, the wife grew up poor and saw her mother struggle to handle the matters of the household. Swearing to create a different type of home for her family, she dedicated herself to being an overachieving super mom.

This mother came to realize that it was she who wasn't giving herself credit for all she did for the family, not her husband. She held an unconscious belief that according to her unrealistic standard, everything she did somehow wasn't enough. In order to compensate, she projected her lack of self-appreciation for what she was doing onto her husband, seeking outer validation from him to alleviate her feelings of guilt and inadequacy from a belief that wasn't true.

Once the unconscious belief is discovered, it's important to practice authentic self-forgiveness. This isn't about forgiving yourself for doing something "wrong" because we're all doing the best we can. You forgive yourself for judging yourself as bad or wrong for what you believe you did or didn't do. The woman in our example might write:

> *I forgive myself for judging myself as inadequate and guilty of failing my family. I recognize the validity of everything I do for my family and appreciate all efforts I make to help others and myself. I am enough.*

Step 5
Outer Treatment

Now it's time to apply your inner work to the outer world. Sometimes just having the information I've shared with you can diffuse much of the volatility from a situation.

In our example, the woman might consider writing nightly in a journal 10 things she appreciated about herself each day. Writing is a powerful door into the subconscious. She might schedule several enjoyable activities she has been wanting to do apart from her family as a way to anchor self-appreciation in her consciousness.

Step 6
Gratitude

It's time to express gratitude for recognizing and taking the opportunity to free yourself from old hurts and false beliefs that were negatively affecting your life and relationships. What was once viewed as a problem turned out to be a gift.

With the false belief gone, there is no longer an unconscious need to project it onto another person and create the same relationship problem again. You are free! It doesn't matter how you do it, just express your gratitude in a way that's meaningful to you.

Step 7
Surrender

You have already done the inner work to heal the issue inside of you that brought you into this difficult situation. If you commit yourself to doing things to anchor your new belief in consciousness, one of two things will happen. Either the other person in your relationship will change their behavior toward you because you have changed or your higher frequency won't be in sync with theirs and they will move out of your life. Either way, it's important to surrender to the fact that whatever happens is for the highest good of both of you.

Symbolic rituals are great for anchoring concepts into our unconscious. Find a relatively smooth rock that can fit in the palm of your hand. With a marker or piece of chalk, write the name of the person involved in your relationship on one side. On the other, write all the emotions you would like to release such as anger, blame, or jealousy. If you are near a body of water such as a pond, lake, stream, or the ocean, take it there and release it.

Don't just toss it in. Take a moment and feel the weight of the rock in your hand as if it's the weight on your heart. Then with a wide swing and the feeling of freedom that comes with it, throw the rock into the water. Feel the lightness in your palm, then hold your palm to your heart.

If you're not near a body of water, dig a small hole and bury the rock. The earth has great transformative powers to break things down and turn them into nourishment. Be sure to sense the feeling of lightness in your hand and heart as well.

Your most important relationship is the one you have with yourself. It's the only one you'll have your entire life. When you understand projections, you'll break unconscious behavioral patterns, make better choices, and know what it's like to be fully in charge of your own happiness.

Like a good wine, from this sweeter position, you'll be able to look back on the bitter times not with regret but with the self-awareness that allows you to say, "It was a very good year."

Chapter 3

Complement Not Conflict

Respecting male and female differences

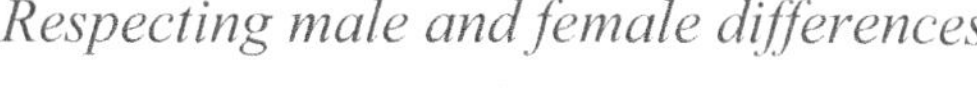

At the level of spirit, there is no sex, sexuality, or duality. In the human experience where the dance of duality creates physical life, masculine and feminine sexual energies influence every part of our existence.

Honoring and working with these different energies is the key to healthy, creative partnerships and satisfying, romantic relationships. Learning to respect both the masculine and feminine energies equally is essential to healing many of the painful issues that plague our society and create violence and destruction worldwide.

The principle of masculine and feminine energy is part of the universal law that governs the world in which we live. We see it all around us in nature. At its most basic level, it controls the expansion and contraction cycles we see throughout the universe.

Look around you and you'll see that nothing is static or stands still. Subatomic particles like protons and electrons pulsate with expansion and contraction. Around 75 times per minute, your heart does the same thing through beating. The tide comes in from the ocean expanding and goes out again by contracting. The foliage of plants and trees expands outward with the summer and retreats with the winter. All participants in the ebb and flow of life conform to this cosmic dance.

Even the circumstances of our lives follow the rhythm of expansion and contraction. Sudden unemployment puts us into a state of depression and contraction whereas winning the lottery launches us into a euphoric state of expansion. While we mistakenly label these experiences good and bad, together they work toward our overall growth. Neither is more beneficial than the other.

Sex is a dance between various states of expansion and contraction. Most people mistake orgasm for the height of expansion whereas it's actually the point of extreme contraction. The height of expansion comes immediately afterward when we collapse into the arms of our partner with an immense feeling of boundlessness and bliss. In that moment there is no you, me, or even time itself. Everything coalesces into the now.

Timeless union is another name for oneness. It's the death of the ego which is why the French have a term for it, *Le Petit Mort* or the little death. This is the moment where we can experience divine union and transcend the physical. Unfortunately, many a man would rather avoid it by rolling over after orgasm, falling asleep, and going back into unconsciousness.

I'm sure you've seen sci-fi movies where a spaceship is preparing to go into hyperspace and travel at warp speed through a wormhole to a distant galaxy light-years away. While the process builds slowly, the ship ultimately finds itself sucked into a vacuum going at a speed that's almost unbearable but soon emerges on the other side into a peaceful, starry cosmos. In sex, orgasm is the supersonic ride through the vacuum, but we can't get to paradise if we back out or blackout before we reach the real destination.

Only when we open ourselves to exploring sex's spiritual nature can we understand that sex alone is physical whereas love is spiritual. Placing the intention of divine union before each sexual encounter, even if it's just a quickie, increases our chances of transcending the state of twoness and entering into the oneness true love makes possible.

The Other Side of Orgasm

Most of us have the idea of love backwards. We think that love comes before sex. In one sense it does, but stay with me as I explain. How many times, predominantly with men but also with women, have we made love the preface to sex only to be disappointed? We convince ourselves we love someone. The thrill of the chase and infatuation keep us pursuing that person right up to the point where we have sex. Soon after, whatever "love" we felt fades away. We used love as a preface for sex. Once sex was achieved, love wasn't needed anymore and neither was our partner.

The good news is real love *does* exist, but it's hiding on the *other* side of the orgasm. When we approach sex as a meditation through orgasm, the love we already have for our partner will be experienced at depths we could never have imagined.

Sexual energy is grounded in the second chakra or body energy center, and all casual sex keeps it locked at that level. This isn't a judgment on casual sex, just something you should know. Not every sexual encounter needs to be mind-blowing or earth-shattering, but if you have lots of sexual encounters with little or no emotional satisfaction, you stunt your ability to create deeper sexual connections by training yourself to not want more. In time, this type of detached sex becomes an unconscious habit. With partners we actually love, the intention should be to raise the level of sexual energy to at least the fourth chakra, the heart, and preferably above.

It's been said that we are not human beings having a spiritual experience but spiritual beings having a human experience. While I believe this to be true, I would add that when we can consciously have a sexual experience as fully empowered spiritual beings, we won't need the pervious part of that statement to remind us of who we really are. The sexual experience alone will make our true spiritual nature self-evident.

Masculine & Feminine Energy

The masculine/feminine dual nature of life has been known for thousands of years. Ancient cultures regarded the sun as masculine and the moon as feminine. The planet Mars is masculine, while Venus is feminine. In astrology, the air and fire signs are masculine whereas the earth and water signs are feminine. We speak of Mother Earth and Father Time. This symbolism represents the relationship between these two primal energies that together animate all of life.

In order for relationships and life to be balanced, equal weight must be given to both of these sexual energies. We all have masculine and feminine energy inside us, and we fluctuate between these energies throughout the day depending on what we're doing.

While some men may exude more feminine energy and some women more masculine energy, on the whole, the majority of men live predominantly in their masculine energy and women in their feminine energy.

I'll be using a heterosexual model to explain these concepts so the points are easily understood, but know that the masculine/feminine interplay of energies applies to all intimate relationships. This dynamic isn't about sex roles but focuses on the ebb and flow of sexual energy between partners. It's about understanding how you hold your sexual energy in any given moment and its effect on your relationship.

When masculine and feminine energies are in their full expression, they are polarized. While there are many different kinds of relationships and reasons why people enter into them, if you seek a high level of attraction and a strong bond in a sexual relationship, the energies the partners carry must be highly polarized. Like magnets, male and female energies attract one another. These ideas have been deeply explored and convincingly presented in the fundamental works of authors Dr. John Gray[1] and David Deida.[2]

An exciting study of more than 1,000 brain scans proves what we have all known intuitively for thousands of years when it comes to the differences in how men and women think. Despite how some may try to deny it, the brains of men and women are wired differently. In the male brain, the neural networks are more concentrated from front to back *within* each hemisphere, making men better at things like spatial relations (determining direction), hand-eye coordination (sports and tool-working), and linear concentration (intense focus on one thing at a time). In contrast, the neural networks of women's brains are more concentrated from side to side *between* hemispheres. This explains why women are generally more socially and emotionally open, good communicators, and multitaskers.[3] At the same time, brain function can differ between men and women so much that artificial intelligence models (AI) can detect whether a scan of brain activity came from a man or woman with greater than 90% accuracy.[4] This difference in brain function is also why women have a more complex sexual arousal process.

Though masculine and feminine energies are different, they exist to *complement* each other, not to *compete* with or change each other. They are not opposing energies but balancing forces that create stability and wholeness. Like two notes in a musical chord or two pieces of a puzzle that interlock to make a complete picture, they are harmonizing energies that work perfectly together if we can allow them to do so.

This difference is beautifully represented in the interlocking teardrop shapes of the ancient Taoist yin-yang symbol or taijitu with the black teardrop representing yin or feminine energy curving around and mutually supporting the white teardrop of masculine or yang energy. Together they create a perfect circle symbolizing balance, oneness, and the divine interplay of nature's primal forces.

Throughout the course of a day men and women can fluctuate between their masculine and feminine energies. Being able to flow between male and female energy in order to accomplish different tasks and experience life is one of the greatest gifts of being human. A man conducting a home repair project is in his masculine energy but stopping to console a child who has had an accident, he switches to his nurturing, feminine energy, but then returns to his masculine energy to finish the project. Likewise, a woman who takes some food to a sick friend is in her feminine energy but at work leading a team training session switches to masculine energy. Back at home for the evening and relaxing in a warm bath, she returns to feminine energy.

While men and women flow between the two sexual energies as needed rather freely, men will instinctively return to masculine energy as their natural state of being and women to feminine energy. Learning to appreciate the gifts of both masculine and feminine energy is essential if a sexual relationship is to be healthy, balanced, and polarized. Relationship bonds start to weaken and lose polarization when women expect their men to be more like women, and men want their women to be more like men. In other words, women want men to like shopping, express their feelings, and be more social, while men want their women to like camping, not be so talkative, and watch more football games. It's long overdue that men and women learn to appreciate their differences and how they were created to support *not mimic* each other because research shows less than two in 10 men and women share personality traits with the opposite sex.[5]

Mars & Venus

The religious myths of Hinduism provide a beautiful metaphor for the dual nature of God with the masculine energy represented by the god Shiva and the feminine energy represented by the goddess Shakti. Shiva and Shakti together represent All-That-Is. Together they are the one, yet they represent the duality we experience as separate souls having a human experience. When these energies are attracted to each other, they bring us back into wholeness.

Shiva is the transcendent aspect of existence, totally free and boundless. It's pure consciousness without form. He holds the potential to become anything. Shakti represents fecundity and is the creative power of the universe. Through her association with Shiva, she manifests form out of pure consciousness. She is the creator, the nurturer, and the protector.

Hindu tradition tells us it is the feminine form of God that dances and attracts Shiva from out of the limitlessness of potential and into the focused energy of creation. Only by bringing their creative energies together are they able to manifest life.

Shakti attracts the masculine through her promise of abundance and the sheer joy of creation. She brings life into being, giving purpose to existence. A woman who embodies her feminine energy invites a man into her heart so that he can experience the fullness of life and the ecstasy of love. A man who is fully inhabiting his masculine energy provides inspiration and activation, helping the feminine to focus her creative energies.

The symbol for the male sex is the circle with an arrow protruding from it. As part of Greco-Roman astronomy, it was shorthand for the planet Mars and sometimes for the god of the same name with the circle representing his shield and the arrow his spear. With this in mind, we can say that masculine energy is directional. It's active energy that sets a goal and moves in the direction to achieve it. It's driven, assertive, and gets things done. Just like Mars, the god of war, masculine energy is ready to conquer the world.

Because of this, women are attracted to men with clear goals to continually improve themselves and move their lives forward personally and professionally. They need to be sure that any man they contemplate being with has the motivation and capability to not only provide a good life for himself but for his future wife and children, as well. Even women with professional positions seek a man who can contribute to the success of their family on equal terms and be a leader in ways that are indicative of a strong husband and father. As such, masculine energy isn't based in having a muscular body or being an athlete, although those things can definitely amplify it. It begins with motivation, goal-setting, and achievement.

Because masculine energy is *doing* energy, not *being* energy, the quickest way to emasculate a man and depolarize a sexual relationship is to criticize the way he's doing something or the direction he has taken. Masculine energy prides itself on solving problems. When a man is criticized for his direction or decision in doing something it's the same as saying, "You're not man enough to handle this." This doesn't mean women can't propose ideas to their men, but it must be done in a way that respects masculine energy's *need to lead* and is not condescending.

If a man is lacking passion or a purpose in life, it's important to do some self-exploration about what matters most to him. Create a specific plan for the future and set incremental goals to realize that vision. While setting goals based on his passion, it's important to engage in activities that provide him with a sense of satisfaction and accomplishment. A man creating something that has a purpose, fills a need, or solves a problem for himself and/or others will strongly engage masculine energy as will improving his body and increasing his physical strength and power.

The Greco-Roman symbol for female or feminine energy is the circle with a cross protruding from it. It represents the planet Venus as well as Aphrodite, the goddess of love. The cross connected to the larger circle is said to be the handle of Aphrodite's hand mirror into which she peers. This represents the introspective and contemplative nature of feminine energy that, unlike masculine energy which is focused on conquering the outside world, is more interested in understanding our internal world. As such, feminine energy is based in emotion, nurturing, compassion, self-reflection, and learning. This is why women make the best teachers and nurses although many men also exist in those professions.

While masculine energy is active, feminine energy is passive but that doesn't mean powerless, far from it. The strength of feminine energy comes from its grounded quality. While masculine energy is like the storm winds that blow over the earth creating great change, feminine energy is like the earth itself, remaining unchanged at its core no matter what happens on the surface. Masculine energy is the power of a fiery speech delivered to a large crowd while feminine energy is the inherent power of a person in deep meditation. Masculine energy seeks to make its power known while feminine energy rests in its power until it's needed.

Because of this, men are attracted to women who can provide the kind of emotional support they need to succeed in their goals and for their family to be grounded in love, nurturing, and emotional wellbeing. A man needs to know his wife believes in him and his plan for their family's future. In fact, her support is crucial to his success. When he can't yet see a way forward, she must be the calm at the center of the storm, providing reassurance to him and her family that everything will be okay in the same way she would comfort a child after an accident.

For a man to express his goals and dreams requires great courage since for masculine energy the greatest fear is failing in life. We see this personified through all the various mythologies of the ages where most stories with a male protagonist involve going out into the world to slay monsters and conquer kingdoms. In this way, a man's drive to conquer the world by realizing his vision and accomplishing his goals is central to his reason for being.

For a man to open his heart and share a risk he is taking requires strength. Don't think for a moment he doesn't lie awake at night thinking, "What if I'm wrong? What if this deal falls through? Is this the right way to expand the business? What if I lose my family's respect?" He knows that if he fails, he's also failing the people he loves the most, his wife and children.

When a man shares his concerns about his goals with his female companion, that's when he depends on her for loving compassion and support. When a woman realizes these aren't just his goals but part of the family's goals, it's easier to be grateful that her man has opened himself to her in this way.

Mutual Support

As with masculine energy, feminine energy is not based in outward appearances. It's not about wearing pretty clothes and makeup. While those things can certainly enhance a woman's feminine energy, it's really about being able to access and exist within the qualities of compassion, support, nurturing, introspection, intuition, and love. It can be difficult for some women to go within and connect to these internal energies when they spend so much of the day inhabiting their masculine energy as leaders, managers, and executives across corporate America. Because women spend so much time expending their energy outward, it can be a challenge to suddenly stop and direct their attention inward.

Women learning to nurture themselves can go a long way toward learning to nurture others. Feminine energy lives in the body and is about sensuality in all its forms. Because of this, a long relaxing bath, massage, spa appointment, or yoga or dance class can help quiet the mind and open the heart to receive nourishing touch and reignite feminine energy. These physical sensations and activities help draw consciousness out of the busy mind and ground it in the body which is where it needs to be for women to be good nurturers. Women often forget to put themselves on their own To Do lists, but when they learn how to properly receive nurturing and know that it's not selfish to do so, they'll be even better at giving it.

Because feminine energy is based in emotion (the heart) and masculine energy is based in intellect (the head) communication between the sexes is often challenging but it doesn't have to be. When we understand our partner's sexual energy and how to accommodate it, communication and mutual support happen more naturally and freely.

Imagine a woman has just had a painful phone conversation with her mother. She seeks out her male partner and begins to tell him about her conversation. While she may cry as she recounts the details of the call, what she's seeking from him is comfort and affirmation, not necessarily an analysis of the conversation or a solution to what her man sees as the problem. The key is to honor her emotional process and provide support without over-analyzing the situation. If her man doesn't listen but dismisses her concerns, patronizes her, or ignores her, he fails her. Whereas a man can be emasculated by a woman's criticism of his need to lead and provide direction, so too can a woman have her femininity diminished by her man's inability to take her feelings seriously. She doesn't need her situation resolved, only to have him listen while she figures out what to do or specifically asks for his advice.

When a woman is accused of being overly emotional, it can trigger feelings of desperation and emotional abandonment. By failing to hold a safe space for his woman's natural expression, a man makes his support unreliable, and his woman feels betrayed by him. In the same way feminine energy works to support a man's leadership and direction, masculine energy works to provide emotional support to the feminine. If a man in his masculine energy cannot be the rock upon which the waves of emotional feminine energy can break and come to rest, the relationship will become depolarized, and she will lose her attraction to him.

Feminine energy feels things deeply, so much so that it can lead women to assume that what they're feeling is glaringly obvious to their male partners. Let me assure you that it isn't. How many times has a woman been upset with her man, thinking he's eventually going to ask her what's wrong when three days later all her pent-up hurt explodes because she thinks he's ignoring her? Naturally, the man is blindsided by her emotional explosion that seems to come out of nowhere. "How am I supposed to read your mind?" he asks in exasperation.

While feminine energy is intuitive and can interpret many of the nonverbal cues and emotional subtext in relationships, it is a mistake to assume masculine energy functions the same way. It does not. Remember, masculine energy is *intellectual*, not emotional, *direct* and not subtle. When women are in conflict with each other, feminine energy takes the battle behind the scenes with subtle attacks on each other like backbiting, spreading rumors, exclusion from social groups, and other passive aggressive actions. When men are in conflict with each other, they deal with it directly. The issue is brought out in the open with one man challenging the other face to face; "You want to step outside and settle this once and for all?"

Because of this vital difference in the way men and women communicate and process emotion and conflict, it's essential that women never assume men know what they're feeling. The best way for a woman to communicate with masculine energy is to express exactly *what* she's feeling and *why* she's feeling it. For example, "I *feel taken for granted* because you agreed we'd go to the business dinner and *expected me to just cancel my existing plans*."

At the same time, women need to say exactly what they're feeling *when* they're feeling it or as soon as it's appropriate to do so. Don't let time go by allowing anger to fester, and when feelings are expressed, never imply or suggest *anything*. To give a man the opportunity to supply the emotional support a woman needs, she has to express her needs in a way that allows him to understand and respond accordingly.

Expressions of Love

Because the concentration of neural networks in men's and women's brains are so different, men can concentrate on a single task with laser-like precision while women are better multitaskers with their attention flowing more freely between activities. A man who is concentrating deeply on a home repair project and is startled by his partner may snap at her unintentionally because the transition in consciousness for him was so jarring. At the same time, a woman will not appreciate her man criticizing her style of organization when he should know she has everything under control even though it may not seem like it to him. Understanding how masculine and feminine attention work differently helps avoid assumptions and unnecessary arguments.

Even so, some men and women still feel disregarded, unloved, or rejected when their partner turns their attention away from them to other activities. These feelings can arise due to unresolved emotional issues from the past resulting in low self-esteem and always needing external attention or affirmation.

Many arguments arise between couples when one or both partners feel unloved. Most often when we feel unloved, *what we are actually experiencing is our own rejection of love.* For feminine energy, love is like water flowing fast and deep with lots of levels, colors, and sensations. For masculine energy, love is like a rock, solid, constant, and unwavering.

To avoid the unnecessary pain of feeling unloved, it's vital to recognize how your partner is *already expressing love* through his or her respective masculine or feminine energy. The ultimate goal should be to transcend the changing flow of emotions in a relationship and concentrate on giving and receiving love through your masculine or feminine energy in each moment. More love—not emotion—in your relationship will deepen the intimacy and strengthen the bond between you.

If you've been in a relationship for a while and have been paying attention, you should be able to recognize how your partner responds to the different ways you give love and extend intimacy. Some people are more receptive to certain kinds of expression than others because there are different ways of showing love.

The revolutionary book *The 5 Love Languages* by Gary Chapman explains that most people prefer to receive love in one or two of five different ways. The five different ways most people express love are through words of affirmation, acts of service, physical affection, quality time, and gifts. When we understand our own love language as well as our partner's, we are better able to prevent feelings of neglect and keep our relationship strong.

Intimacy won't get lost in translation because each partner has learned to speak the other's love language. Understanding how your partner prefers to be loved will definitely increase the intimacy in your relationship. For example, a woman may find that her husband is less responsive to the little unexpected gifts she gives him but is truly touched and grateful when she does something for him that makes his day easier like mowing the backyard. This is because since masculine energy is *doing* energy, it more easily recognizes acts of service as an expression of love. In contrast, understanding the emotional basis of feminine energy, many women would more readily respond to physical affection and words of affirmation.

Of course, for a woman it also helps to see how her man is *already* expressing his love for her and their family through masculine energy by providing for them financially, establishing a home, protecting them, investing for their future, conducting home repairs, and so on. At the same time, it's important for a man to acknowledge his female partner's expressions of love through her feminine energy by the way she touches his hand in the car, cares for their children, supports his vison for their future, and such. When men and women can recognize all the masculine and feminine expressions of love that *already exist in their relationship* and can express gratitude for them, neither will feel neglected or unloved.

Different Experiences of Sex

In sex, the male must hold all the masculine energy and the female must fully embody her feminine energy or the passion will fade. It can be hard for a female civil engineer who has been leading a large team all day to relax back into her feminine energy in the evening or a male child psychologist who has been comforting children all day to fully reconnect with his masculine energy. Even so, it's vital that both partners be able to recalibrate back into their inherent sexual energies through some of the ways we discussed earlier in order for the polarization and sexual desire to remain strong.

For the most part, sex is an external, pleasure-based experience for men and an internal, emotion-based experience for women. A man's sex organs are all outside his body whereas a woman's sex organs are predominantly internal. Sex takes place inside her body and outside of his. It is she who must become vulnerable and open herself to him. He doesn't have to do that. Intercourse takes place inside her body and outside of his. These physical metaphors explain much about why men and women view and experience sex so differently. Neither view is right or wrong. It just is.

Men have traditionally treated sex like a great steak that will still taste good no matter what kind of day they've had or mood they're in. Emotion doesn't play a large role in the experience. This isn't an insult just a real-world observation that wouldn't offend most men. Women need to understand that men aren't being callous or intentionally distant during sex. It's how masculine energy and their physiology are constructed.

To generate more intimacy in the bedroom, it helps to start cultivating intimacy outside the bedroom. As a woman, when you reach across the car seat and touch your man's hand, intimacy is created and words are unnecessary. The next time you kiss him, try cupping his cheek in the palm of your hand at the same time. Touching someone's face creates a deep sense of intimacy. If his tie is crooked, offer to straighten it for him and let your hands run down his chest as you smooth his shirt. These are small actions, but they build intimacy in powerful ways by subtly drawing a man's consciousness out of his head and into his body.

There is no magic bullet here. Even so, both man and woman will get less frustrated in all aspects of their relationship if they remember how masculine and feminine energy work. When it comes to men and sex, they aren't trying to hurt or disappoint their women, and they certainly aren't rejecting them. Energetically and spiritually, a man is drawn to a woman because he's looking to her for wholeness. He needs her to help him open to intimacy by guiding him into his heart through a deeper connection to his body.

Chapter 4

Abiding Intimacy

Why we crave deep connection

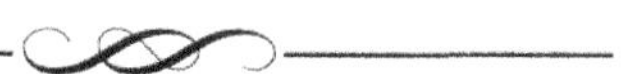

When two people come together in a romantic relationship, the purpose is to be as one, creating and abiding in intimacy. It's said that we live, move, and have our being in God. What is God but unity and wholeness? It is only within wholeness where we find unconditional love because there is no distinction between one and the other. True intimacy is the closest we can come to manifesting the presence of God in our human lives, and marriage is the formal commitment to achieving that state of being.

At a certain point along our spiritual path, my wife Sherry and I made the decision to become ordained ministers. We did so because we felt a calling to be of service to others on a deeper level. At first, we didn't make the fact of our ordination widely known. As word slowly got out, we began to receive requests from friends and colleagues to perform their wedding ceremonies. We usually perform them together. When we do, one of the spiritual gifts we focus on is intimacy.

A great example of intimacy involves the life of renowned architect and philosopher Buckminster Fuller. The bond between Fuller and his wife, Anne, was a strong one, so much so that people often commented on how much in love they seemed to be. In 1983 after 66 years of marriage, Fuller sat at his wife's bedside holding her hand with his head bowed as she lay dying in a coma. After being left alone for some time with his wife, his children reentered the room to find Fuller in the same position over an hour later. Fuller had passed away, and within hours Anne would join him.

When two people who have loved each other over half a century make their transition from this life at virtually the same time, especially when one of them is perfectly healthy, it isn't a coincidence. There are many such stories. To me, they are the truest and most beautiful examples of intimacy where two people really have become one.

Coalescing & Craving

There is a wonderful scientific principle that demonstrates this idea perfectly. It's called critical proximity. Automaker Henry Ford was looking to create a new method to document the measurements for the manufacture of auto parts in a way that was far more precise than anything available in the late 19th century. Swedish machinist Carl Edvard Johansson was hired as the contractor and created what's known today as gauge blocks. These ceramic or metal measuring blocks are precision-ground to such a fine degree that there are absolutely no irregularities or differences on their perfectly straight surfaces. Because of this, they can detect length differences as small as one ten-thousandth of an inch.

To measure various lengths, the blocks cannot simply be placed one on top of the other. They have to be slid together. When this happens, there is less than one molecule of atmosphere between their ultra-flat, perfectly smooth surfaces. This makes it impossible to pull them apart. They are two and yet one at the same time. Measurements with gauge blocks need to be made quickly because the atoms within them are now in critical proximity. In a short period of time, they will coalesce into one single piece of metal or ceramic again.

This is what Sherry and I mean when we speak of intimacy. Like making gauge blocks, it's about grinding off all the misunderstandings, misidentifications, and misinterpretations from our consciousness so that we can coalesce with our partners and thus with God in a spiritual union by returning to our true essence of oneness.

As previously discussed, we have three aspects of ourselves only one of which represents who we really are. These are the person we *think* we are and present to the world, our *unconscious mind*, and our *essential self*. The spiritual work we do on ourselves is the polish we place on the surface of our souls that will allow us to coalesce back into our loving essence, back into God and finally back into the divinely satisfying intimate relationship with another person which we all crave.

While intimacy in oneness is the most satisfying part of a relationship, it doesn't necessarily require two people to achieve it. Because God is everywhere and in all things, we can choose to coalesce with divine consciousness in many ways. Sherry and I often lose ourselves in a beautiful walk in nature, during meditation, while dancing, or when listening to music. As the ancient poet Rumi said, it's in these moments that we remove all that is not loving about ourselves and converge with God who is only love.

Defining the Indefinable

If oneness through intimacy is a natural part of our being, why doesn't this degree of love happen more often? Why do these amazing stories about couples like Buckminster Fuller and his wife always seem like the exception rather than the rule?

Perhaps it's because we've never really known how to define the indefinable state of intimacy. While writing this book, I was looking through a thesaurus for synonyms for the word intimacy. I found words like understanding, closeness, caring, affection, tenderness, and warmth. We can have friendships with closeness and caring, but to me this isn't intimacy. We often show affection, tenderness, and warmth to our pets, but that isn't intimacy either. It seemed strange to me that in the enormous lexicon of the English language, the state of being and kind of relationship we're all pursuing has no additional descriptors. Perhaps this lack of defining terms and misunderstanding explains why so many relationships fail. It may also be the reason we go from partner to partner searching for the ineffable essence we can't quite describe or identify but that we all know intuitively is essential to our wellbeing.

Intimacy is an almost ethereal concept like God. While we can't say specifically what it is, we know it's real when we *feel* it. Like God, intimacy resides within us and isn't something we get from another person. It's a state of consciousness we choose to inhabit.

Science has clearly shown that everything in existence, from human beings to a supernova a thousand light-years away, is made of exactly the same thing—energy. To be in a state of divine consciousness is to operate from the perspective that we are all one. I mean this *literally*. You are a manifestation of divine energy expressing itself in human form as you journey through life, the purpose being to learn and grow from experiences as only *you* create them. The same goes for me and everyone else who has ever lived.

When we realize that our names and seemingly separate personalities are just temporary masks we wear and our life stories are just scripts we're writing and playing out for a short 70 or more years, we can detach from the world of duality. We can escape the false paradigm of me/you and us/them and live in a state of wholeness where all that exists is the divine union. This is what intimacy is all about.

There's a simple Sanskrit mantra called So Hum that means *I am that*. During meditation, *So* (I am) is said mentally on the inhale while *Hum* (that) is thought on the exhale. It's a reminder that, on a spiritual level, you are everything and everyone you see. This gives real and literal meaning to the phrase, "Do unto others as you would have them do unto you." Choose your words and actions wisely because the only recipient of your deeds is *you*. Without this realization, the best we can achieve in a relationship is the temporary satiation of our physical needs and emotional deficiencies.

What Intimacy Is Not

The idea that sex equals intimacy comes from the assumption that sexual intercourse is the closest we can ever get to another human being or the closest two human beings can ever come to merging into one entity. While this may be true from a physical standpoint, the body isn't who we are. If the consciousness of the participants doesn't merge at the same time, then all you're left with is physical stimulation and not divine unification.

Relationships fall apart not because of a lack of physical stimulation. A person can get that almost anywhere. Whether they know it or not, it's the lack of deep connection that causes someone to seek unity elsewhere. When people are unfaithful in their marriage, their partners immediately become insecure thinking their spouses strayed because the other man or woman is younger, better looking, has a better body, or makes more money. In most cases, it's none of those things. A woman who had an affair once said she did so not because of how her lover looked but how he *made her feel*. Not making excuses for her infidelity, that response signaled there was lack of intimacy in her marriage for quite some time before the affair.

We also make the mistake of assuming intimacy is emotion. Lots of women complain that their husband or boyfriend isn't emotionally available. We've already talked about how masculine and feminine energy experience emotions differently and how those differences should be respected and accommodated to strengthen a relationship. Intimacy isn't the ability to express emotion. Many relationships have lots of emotion flying around and we call it drama.

For two people to really come together it requires setting aside the self we present to the world and falsely believe ourselves to be. Intimacy requires *empathy*, not emotion. When we can put ourselves in the place of someone else and feel what they are going through as if it were our own experience, our spirits are merging in a deeply intimate way. We are residing in divine consciousness and living in oneness.

Divine Mandate

Subconsciously, our ravenous spiritual hunger drives us to merge with God, our source, through uniting with the God essence in each other. This is what we really yearn for in intimate relationships. We find our home in the presence of being understood completely and loved unconditionally. Why? It's because when it comes to God consciousness, we are a part of it on one hand while on the other we embody the whole of it.

Most of us have heard the phrase "two becoming one" so many times that it either passes through our minds completely unnoticed or we view it as an unattainable cliché. If any long-term relationship is to survive and thrive, real intimacy attained by becoming one is the next step. It's critical to human evolution and the real reason people couple. The reason isn't to have children. The entire animal kingdom procreates just fine without intimacy and with only a few exceptions doesn't practice monogamy either.

Human beings are drawn together in pairs and seek lifetime unions because we have a higher mandate that involves expanding divine consciousness through spiritual union. Intimacy requires each person to merge into something greater than themselves. The ego can falsely perceive this as a death and fight vehemently to maintain its sense of separateness. This is what's meant by the ancient statement that we must lose our life if we wish to save it. It takes courage to let go and become one.

Both parties in a relationship must recognize themselves within the other in order for intimacy to be achieved. A drop of sea water returned back into the ocean immediately recognizes itself as part of the whole and merges joyfully and completely. In contrast, a drop of oil that is entirely different in its makeup remains separate on the surface of the water and never assimilates for a deeper experience.

For those struggling with intimacy issues, the best thing to do is to cultivate divine consciousness through meditation or an activity like yoga, Tai Chi, or Qigong that requires letting go, release of the ego, and surrender to a force greater than ourselves.

To commune with another in the presence of God, we must be able to create our own intimate relationship with God. In this way, we will be able to commune with God in others, no longer needing to define the indefinable because we will have experienced it for ourselves.

Chapter 5

In Sync with Healing

How sex aligns the body for health

Scientific research has only recently begun to uncover an obscure and largely disregarded nerve in the brain that appears to have the power to synchronize a host of biological systems and realign the body for health. When properly activated, it's showing great potential to fight disease and bring the rest of the body back online. Even more interesting, it's related to sexual functions.

Medicine has known of the cranial nerves since at least 250 AD. These nerves emerge from the bottom of the brain in pairs and govern major functions of the body. They are numbered 1 through 12 beginning with those closest to the forehead. Among their functions is providing for the vital senses of smell, sight, hearing, taste, and touch as well as movement of the eyes, tongue, jaw, and face. Cranial Nerve 1 is the olfactory nerve that branches to the nose and governs the sense of smell while Cranial Nerve 2 is the optic nerve managing sight, and so on.

Discovery Dismissed

It was in 1878 that German scientist Gustav Fritsch detected a new cranial nerve in the brain of a shark. It was at the front just before Cranial Nerve 1, the olfactory nerve, running parallel to it. It was much thinner than the other nerves and could be easily missed if a person wasn't looking for it, but its presence was unmistakable.

The existence of a 13th cranial nerve seemed preposterous to the medical establishment and its reality was quickly dismissed. It was believed by anatomists back then, as well as today, that the reason the 13th cranial nerve was missing in brains used in medical research was because it was inadvertently removed along with the tough coverings of the brain during dissection. Even so, scientists who believed in the 13th cranial nerve's existence didn't know how to categorize it in their studies. In reality, the new nerve should have been classified Cranial Nerve 1 because it emerged first in the brain ahead of the olfactory nerve, but the existing 12 cranial nerves were too entrenched in medical history and literature to renumber all of them at that point. As such, it was decided the classification for the new cranial nerve would be Cranial Nerve Zero or CN0 sometimes called the terminal nerve.

Even today, the presence of CN0 is still debated. Most doctors aren't aware of it because it doesn't appear in any medical textbooks. This is in spite of the fact that Fritsch's discovery had been found in the brains of nearly all vertebrates and in humans by 1913.

Sexual Suggestions

Like the olfactory nerve, CN0 is closely tied to the nose. If CN0 were involved in our general sense of smell, it would feed back into the olfactory bulb, a massive cluster of synapses with odor receptors for 347 different kinds of scents, but it doesn't do that. We already have CN1, the olfactory nerve, for that job. It's clear CN0 is doing something very different that also involves our sense of smell.

All the evidence we have about CN0 strongly suggests that its function involves subliminal sexual attraction by transferring signals from pheromones received in the nasal cavities to the brain.[1] What makes CN0 different is that instead of being anchored in the region of the brain that involves smell, it bypasses the olfactory bulb and sends its signals to the areas of the brain that deal with sexual reproduction. These include the lateral septal nuclei and pre-optic areas that deal with things like the release of hormones and other primal urges such as thirst and hunger.

Humans are part of the animal kingdom. Many animals rely on smell to determine sex, social rank, territories, find reproductive partners, and identify their sexual mates or family members. It's believed this process is facilitated by signals from pheromones that are processed in a vomeronasal organ, a cluster of receptors inside the nasal cavity near the olfactory bulb. Pheromone exposure in animals has been shown to cause a flood of sex hormones into the blood as well as influence estrus, sexual behavior, and ovulation. Humans, however, do not have a vomeronasal organ in the nasal cavity and yet, all the same changes happen to us when exposed to pheromones. It can only be CN0 that is carrying those signals back to the brain and initiating such reactions. We know this for a host of reasons not the least of which is that the activation of CN0 releases a powerful surge of the sex hormone gonadotropin-releasing hormone (GnRH) into the bloodstream.

Activation & Order

It's clear CN0 is involved in sexual response through picking up signals from pheromones and transferring them to the brain, triggering a number of sexual and hormonal changes in the body. Even so, how does this process put the body back in sync for better health?

When CN0 is activated, GnRH is released, acting as the catalyst for other important hormonal changes. Eventually, this leads to the sex act and orgasm during which an intense release of the hormone oxytocin takes place. Known as the "love" hormone, oxytocin generates an intense sense of bonding between two people. Oxytocin also surges during childbirth to bond mother to child and to a slightly lesser degree during breastfeeding.

As CN0 is activated and oxytocin is increased, this process sets off a chain reaction that synchronizes all the other 12 cranial nerves and their related functions. The euphoric state experienced during oxytocin exposure takes the body out of fight-or-flight mode and shifts its functioning from the sympathetic nervous system to the parasympathetic while bringing the hypothalamic-pituitary-adrenal (HPA) axis back online.

At the same time, all functions governed by the autonomic nervous system improve, including heart regulation, blood pressure, clotting capability, and production of immunoglobulin along with many others. Neurotransmitter function improves, norepinephrine, epinephrine, histamine, and melatonin levels normalize while sex hormones are regulated properly and production of natural killer cells improves among other countless benefits. The bottom line is that when CN0 is synchronized so is everything else, and that's what we call *health.*

An additional benefit of CN0 activation and synchronization with the other 12 cranial nerves is that it aligns Cranial Nerve 10 or CN10 also known as the vagus nerve. As the longest cranial nerve in the body, CN10 runs from the brain to the colon. Along the way, it stimulates the muscles of the heart and is deeply involved in the resting heart rate. As such, synchronization of CN0 affects the vagal tone or heart-rate-to-breathing-rate ratio. According to Fredrickson, people with a higher vagal tone experience more moments of positivity resonance because the vagus nerve connects the brain to the heart. They smile more, make more eye contact, have better relationships, and are generally more loving. In this way, CN0 synchronization helps recalibrate the vagal tone automatically, and connecting with others happens more naturally.

Whether it's healing our bodies or healing our relationships, CN0 synchronization is proving to be a powerful tool in recreating our lives. As science continues to reveal more of its healing power, particularly as it relates to oxytocin and certain cancers, CN0 is destined to become an essential modality for total body balancing, synchronization, and a return to health.

In the past, the health benefits of sex were only anecdotally reported, their effect limited to better circulation and the number of calories burned during intercourse. Today, research is showing that oxytocin via CN0 activation and orgasm holds much greater potential to return the body to a healthy state.

The existence of a master cranial nerve like CN0 can no longer be ignored. In short, synchronization of the autonomic nervous system via CN0 activation is the basis of all good health. For this reason, it's long overdue that the medical establishment begin discussing sex as a medical intervention for treating illness and as a pathway to harness the healing power of oxytocin for specific diseases.

Chapter 6

Invisible Attachments

Couples bond by sharing intimate spaces

It wasn't long ago the National Association of Home Builders predicted 60% of all upscale custom-built homes would soon have dual master suites for married couples.[1] To help sell the idea, everyone from marriage counselors to real estate agents was talking about the advantages. No more putting up with your spouse's snoring. Gone were concerns about disturbing the sleep of a partner who worked non-traditional hours. Want to watch TV in bed until 2:00 a.m.? Fine. It was claimed that by making mutual nudity exposure less frequent, separate bedrooms maintained an element of desire and mystery in relationships.[2]

It certainly sounds luxurious and it might be fun to try for a while, but is giving couples more time away from each other the answer to increasing intimacy? The sex might be better at first, but are couples gaining convenience while weakening the connection between them through spending even less time together?

For the majority of Americans, dual master suites aren't an option but a similar home amenity is and it comes with the same pros and cons, It's the trend of having separate his-and-her bathrooms in the master suite. Many couples swear by them. No more dealing with her cosmetic tubes and jars cluttering the countertop. He's a slob but can drop his underwear any place he wants now. The days of crashing into each other during the morning rush to get ready for work are over. Privacy and peace are had at last.

Unfortunately, this convenience can come with a cost. When I first met Windsor Smith, interior designer and author of *Homefront: Design for Modern Living*, at a dinner party, this very subject came up. Ms. Smith, who specializes in designing upscale estates for powerful people, said that in her observation whenever a couple opts for separate bathrooms it usually leads to separate houses and eventually divorce. Could it really be that spending less time together, even under the same roof, is damaging to the strength of relationships?

Logistics aside, sharing the intimate spaces of the home with our partners keeps us bonded to them in ways that are primal to our biology. Invisible forces are at work continually reinforcing our unconscious sense of belonging and attachment to them. Nowhere does this bonding happen to the degree that it does in close communal spaces like the bedroom and bathroom.

Bathroom Bonding

Most working couples scramble through their hectic morning routine trying to get themselves and their children, if any, out the door on time. Late work nights or afterwork errands usually mean many couples and families don't have dinner together anymore either. It seems the last opportunity busy couples have for making a real connection with each other is during their evening routine, usually in the bathroom.

In a recent poll, 45% of the couples responding said they share their nighttime routine with their partner in the bathroom as a way to wind down and talk about the day. This was in contrast to 29% who said they were still able to eat dinner together. For the under 34 crowd, just 16% said they could manage eating dinner together and felt that bathroom bonding was an important way to keep from growing apart.[3]

A great way to deepen this kind of experience might be for each person to participate in some aspect of their partner's nighttime routine. No, you're not going to brush your wife's teeth, but brushing her hair for her before she puts it up or sets it is a loving thing to do while she talks about what's on her mind. Although it might sound impractical, mutual grooming is a high bonding activity in the animal kingdom of which we are a part. Even something as simple as applying lotion to your partner's body and showering together provide the same benefit.

Signature Scents

While the bathroom bonding is in progress, unseen forces are at work increasing intimacy on a subconscious level that can deepen our connection to each other even when we're not together. When we share intimate spaces like a bathroom or bedroom, we're constantly taking in the scent of our partners. Put on your partner's bathrobe because yours is in the laundry and suddenly you're smelling their scent. As far as your nose is concerned, they're practically in the room. Our sense of smell has a strong connection to memory. Thoughts of our partners can enter our minds at times like these further strengthening our connection to them. Post-workout clothes thrown on the bed, hair caught in a brush on the counter, a spouse's pillowcase, and even a shared towel give off olfactory cues that are deepening the bond between us and our partners all the time whether we know it or not.

Although science has never officially determined that each human has an individual scent, police and trailing dogs have been proving it anecdotally for decades. A study performed at University College in London in 1955 proved that dogs could even detect the difference in scent between identical twins. Although the source of human scent wasn't the subject of the study, the researchers inferred that whatever it was, it was probably genetic.[4]

Science is beginning to suspect the unique chemical composition of sebum is what gives us our individual scent.[5] Produced by the sebaceous glands, sebum is a fatty substance that helps lubricate the skin. It is liquid at body temperature and solid at room temperature. Chemically speaking, sebum is made up of fatty acids, wax alcohols, sterols, terpenoids, and hydrocarbons. Some of these compounds aren't found anywhere else in the body. If sebum is removed from the skin, the sebaceous glands work quickly to replace it. That's why dogs can still identify someone's scent even after a vigorous shower or a series of showers.

A structure similar to cholesterol called squalene is also found in sebum. It's the component that helps dogs and other animals distinguish us as different from their own species. It's estimated that unique combinations of fatty acid components and wax alcohols in squalene are what differentiate one human's scent from another.[6]

Just to give you an idea of how individual scent bonds people together, studies using T-shirts worn over several days showed that not only can people detect their own scent, they can identify those of family members, as well.[7] Babies only a few weeks old have shown that they can identify the breast scent of their own mother over those of other mothers.[8] Likewise, mothers can also recognize the scent of their own baby.[9]

Attachment Beyond Awareness

Sharing our intimate spaces with our partners allows for another powerful chemical transfer to take place, the exchange of pheromones. Like human scent, the actual existence of human pheromones and our ability to detect them hasn't been officially demonstrated by science. Most of the issue lies in the fact that other mammals have a special organ to sense pheromones called a vomeronasal organ which humans lack.

When pheromones are in the air, a bundle of nerves in the vomeronasal organ sends messages to the brain that excites the hypothalamus, which controls many functions, including aspects of parenting and attachment. A fairly recent study showed that the hypothalamus of women lit up when exposed to 4,16-androstadien, a synthetic steroid or pherine with male pheromone-like properties.[10]

Since the late 1990s, a mountain of evidence has been building demonstrating that humans probably do have a vomeronasal organ and that it's most likely connected to the nasal septum. At this point, searching for the existence of pheromones is like trying to discover what wind looks like. Even though we can't see it, we can clearly see its effects all around us, which is proof of its reality.

Unlike sebum which adheres to the skin, pheromones are projected into the environment by our bodies. When we're sharing a bathroom or bedroom with our partner, we're giving off these signals all the time. Androstadienone is a prominent steroid hormone in men believed to contain pheromones. It's most prevalent on the skin and hair under the arms and in semen. Several studies have shown that when heterosexual women and homosexual men are exposed to androstadienone, it heightens arousal,[11] alters cortisol levels,[12] and promotes a positive mood state.[13] This is why a synthetic form of androstadienone in the form of a nasal spray is currently being developed for women with social anxiety problems.[14]

Androstadienone exposure for heterosexual women also alters the length and timing of the menstrual cycle, affecting fertility.[15] Women are so sensitive to masculine scents that they can detect exaltolide, a male musk-like compound, at dilutions 1,000 times lower than men.[16] Some researchers feel this high sensitivity to smell aids women in choosing a better mate because they have more invested in the act of procreation.

Likewise, a powerful steroid hormone called estratetraenol is thought to contain pheromones. Found predominantly in female urine, it increases arousal[17] and elevates mood[18] in heterosexual men. In addition, distinct activity in the hypothalamus area of the brain, which is involved in bonding and attachment in heterosexual women and homosexual men, is detected when exposed to androstadienone. The same activity occurs in the brains of heterosexual men as well as homosexual women when exposed to estratetraenol.[19] [20] [21]

The point to all this science is that there is a physiological and chemical connection to our intimate partners going on just beyond our awareness. It's strengthened when we share our intimate spaces with each other because, like the rest of the animal kingdom, we leave our scent everywhere. This "marking" of territory subconsciously confirms to the brains of both partners that *you belong to me.*

When we think about how these invisible chemical connections and communications keep us bonded together on a very real but subconscious level, we have to ask if we've become too clean? The impulse to disinfect everything these days, especially in the bathroom, might be blocking the important chemical messages we are supposed to be receiving from our partners. Maybe some simple soap and water would do instead of a caustic drugstore cleaner. It might be a good idea to reconsider highly fragranced colognes as well as hair and skincare products that can also disrupt the scented signal we're getting from our mates.

Kissing & Connection

Several times each year, my wife Sherry and I conduct a series of nine workshops called the Couples Transformational Intensive which is designed to reduce conflict, increase bonding, and bring intimate partners closer together. One of the simplest but most powerful parts of the program is when couples commit to kissing for five consecutive minutes each day. The kissing doesn't have to lead to sexual activity. If it does, that's fine. The main goal is to make a consistent physical connection every day.

Kissing strengthens the connection between people but especially intimate partners. The lips contain an enormous amount of touch receptors and sebaceous glands. When we kiss, we exchange sebum that contains our unique self-identifying chemical signature along with countless proteins and hormones at homeopathic levels.

Research continues to show that the exchange of sebum most likely plays a prominent role in feelings of attachment both between intimate partners, as well as parents and children.[22] This is why it's instinctual to want to kiss those we love. We want to strengthen the bond between us and them, creating a sort of chemical Wi-Fi that keeps us connected even when we aren't together. I call this invisible bond psycho-spiritual "interraintment," and it's crucial to maintaining the mindset of *two becoming one* in a marriage because that's what these tiny but extremely powerful chemicals do for us on an unconscious level.

From this simple exercise, our workshop couples regularly report dramatic improvements in their relationships that parallel much of the research that has been done on consistent kissing. A recent study followed couples that committed to increasing their daily kissing over a six-week period. Results showed the couples experienced statistically significant decreases in stress and cholesterol levels. This was accompanied by a marked increase in relationship satisfaction.[23]

Nobel Prize-winning scientist Luc Montagnier has scientifically demonstrated that a substance, although diluted thousands of times in water, still remains chemically potent and active. This supports the efficacy of things like homeopathic medicine which uses microscopic doses of substances to heal. It also shows how infinitesimally small amounts of sebum and pheromones can have such a powerful effect on us. Montagnier's research went on to show that even when the original substance couldn't be detected in the water anymore, its electromagnetic signals were still present which produced dramatic biological effects.[24] Maybe it's time to start taking more baths together?

Making the Most of It

Sharing a bathroom or bedroom might not work for all couples, but I urge you to either stick with it or return to it using some of our suggestions. Our primal chemical bonds exist for a reason, and we need to consciously use them to our advantage to keep our modern relationships intact even as the demands of life give us less time together. Quality of time more so than quantity is what will strengthen the busy 21st century relationship, and a shared bathroom has much to offer if you know how to use it.

This might be difficult if your bathroom is the size of a broom closet, but do what you can with what you have. If possible, consider expanding your bathroom. Not only will this improve the value of your home, but you'll naturally want to spend more time pampering yourself and your partner in a larger, more modernized bathroom.

In sharing the bathroom, always set rules concerning your comfort level. If you don't like pop-ins while you're on the toilet, say so. This supports privacy and respect in a relationship, but you might want to leave the door unlocked during your shower in case your partner wants to slip in and surprise you.

It's nice to dream about having a big house and lots of things with which to fill it, but the truth is that big houses and their dual master suites and bathrooms take us further away from each other when we are supposed to be social animals. There's also no more need to compromise or to try to work things out when you have his versus her domains of the house. A lot of the time, this just leads to isolation and narcissism.

When I hear people say that they just fell out of love with someone, I often wonder what really happened. Did they really just lose that loving feeling, or did they lose their unseen loving connection?

Chapter 7

Sex During Pregnancy

What's okay and when?

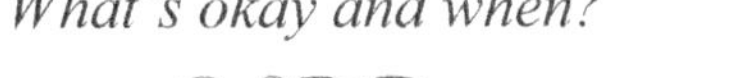

Pregnancy for couples is a wonderful time, especially if it's the first time. There is a lot of excitement but also apprehension about how their lives will change over the next nine months and especially after the baby is born. One of the biggest areas of concern is usually sex during pregnancy. Is it okay? Does it increase the risk of miscarriage? Are there certain positions that should be avoided?

Normal & Natural

Sex is perfectly natural during pregnancy. Penetration cannot harm the baby which is protected by the mother's abdomen, muscular walls of the uterus, and the cushioning of the amniotic sac fluid. The contractions of orgasm cannot trigger the contractions of labor because they're two different biological processes.

Some doctors may ask women to refrain from sex in the final weeks of pregnancy as a precaution against pre-term birth because it's thought that hormones in semen known as prostaglandins can stimulate contractions. This idea arises from the fact that the gel doctors apply to the cervix to induce contractions contains prostaglandins. On the contrary, doctors have encouraged sex for pregnant women who are overdue for this very reason. Keep in mind that the connection between prostaglandins and contractions is only theoretical, and most couples have satisfying sex through the full pregnancy without incident.

Reasons to Abstain

There are times when sex during pregnancy isn't advised. Doctors may recommend refraining from sex if the mother has a history of miscarriages or is experiencing early contractions (before 37 weeks). Unexplained vaginal bleeding, discharge or cramping, and amniotic fluid leakage are all reasons a doctor may recommend refraining from sex. This may also be the case if the cervix has opened too early, the placenta is too low in the uterus, or when the mother is expecting twins, triplets, or more.

Keep in mind that when a doctor recommends no sex it very well may mean no sexual activity, including oral sex that could lead to arousal. Ask questions and be specific.

Position Possibilities

Sexual desire for the woman will ebb and flow during pregnancy, possibly in different ways than she is used to so it's important for her partner to be understanding. There are no sexual positions that are off limits, but preferences may change for comfort reasons as the pregnancy progresses. Avoiding the missionary position after the fourth month may be a good idea. Otherwise, the weight of the baby might create discomfort and constrict major blood vessels. Side-by-side positions or those with the woman on top might work best heading into the third trimester.

Time for Healing

Sexual desire may naturally decrease in the postpartum period (six weeks) after birth. This can be caused by a number of things, including healing from incisions due to episiotomy or cesarean section, fatigue, normal postpartum bleeding, breast tenderness, hormonal fluctuations, or emotional issues from postpartum anxiety. Most doctors will recommend refraining from sex for six weeks after the baby's birth to allow time for healing and to resolve any of these issues. The most important thing is to resume sex when the mother feels emotionally and physically ready to do so.

Chapter 8

Making It Last

Advice from couples married 50 years or more

Every couple goes into marriage with the intent to stay together for a lifetime. Unfortunately, that doesn't happen for many people. The good news, however, is that the overall divorce rate has been dropping since the 1990s and the 50% divorce rate isn't true anymore. What has remained consistent is that two-thirds of all divorces are still initiated by women, especially the late life divorce, the only category that's still rising.[1]

Although many counselors have their own ideas about how to make marriage last, the real experts are the couples who have already made it to 50 years of marriage and beyond. We've all heard long-time married couples attribute their longevity to things like communication, not letting fights last, having a sense of humor, and spending time together. While these are certainly very important parts of keeping a relationship strong over decades, these couples had something different to say to help us think about relationships in a different way.

Don't second guess love

"My grandkids won't settle down because they think the grass is greener. I met my wife and asked her to marry me three days later. When you know someone is right for you, settle down with them and don't let them go. The grass is never greener than love you foster over many years."[2]

—Sheldon Y., 69

Expect there will be hard times

"I got married at age 18. Back then, it was just what you did. At first, it was fun and easy. Then we had one kid, two kids, three kids, four kids. Things got hard. We grew up together and we stayed together as our kids grew up. The secret is that it is hard. When you realize that, you are on track to having a marriage that is filled with love."[3]
—Linda P., 68

Focus on the positive

"We only remember the good times. Learning from bad experiences is important but then we put them away. Focusing on the joyful memories in our relationship gives us the motivation to keep moving forward and the belief that we can create more of them."
—Richard K., 74

Children make marriage stronger

"I've never been sorry for raising the kids when we were young. Now, we're fortunate that our kids all live within 30 minutes of us so we can have get-togethers often."[4]
—Jean T., 73

Talk to each other; don't vent to friends

"People, in my belief, get too much advice and generally the wrong advice. Other people just tie your problems up in knots and make them bigger. It's best to work things out among yourselves."[5]
—Dan T., 77

Give each other personal space

"I credit still being married to living in a big house. I need space. I need to know that I can be by myself and [have room to be] artistic. Tom is happy with 10 books a week in a leather chair."[6]
—Maureen M., 80

Marriage isn't always 50/50

"I had lots of kids and people over all the time…I don't think he's always been totally comfortable … but he put up with it."[7]

—Sharon B., 72

Never stop showing affection

"If you continue holding hands and you're content, that's what's important. Is the sex going to be what it was when you first got married? No, it changes and is replaced with things just as satisfying and fulfilling."

—Evelyn B., 73

Don't let friendships fade

"When you're stuck indoors with a couple of toddlers, a moan on the phone to a friend can stop you taking it out on your partner when he gets home."

—Carol J., 81

Give in occasionally instead of giving up

"If you just can't settle on something—especially if one person is irrational about something and won't budge—that's when what we call give-and-take can be a marriage saver. Give-and-take means first one person in the marriage gives while the other person takes, then vice versa in turns, on and on and on."[8]

—Sonny S., 78

Show respect

"Always make eye contact when listening to your spouse even if you're in the middle of doing something because it respects their thoughts."[9]

—Bill T., 75

There is no secret

"There is no secret. Marriage is hard work. If you want it to work out, you have to not give up on it. Younger people these days think they can get whatever they want when they want it. Marriage doesn't work like that. It takes years to understand a person and it takes guts

to stick with them even when things are not working out as easily as they used to."[10]
—Joe P., 71

Chapter 9

Confrontation Without Conflict

Disagreements don't have to devolve into drama

"If you think you are enlightened, go home for Thanksgiving." With that humbling advice, it's refreshing to know that even spiritual teachers like Ram Dass aren't above being irritated by people who know how to push their buttons. I guess gurus are human after all.

While that's comforting to know, emotional and spiritual growth isn't about getting along with everyone all the time. There will always be a partner, co-worker, boss, parent, sibling or in-law that rubs us the wrong way. The key to reducing the drama in these kinds of relationships isn't to convince the other person that we're right or to change them in any way but to understand ourselves better and why we're allowing these situations to trigger us. When we do, we can consciously navigate these challenging relationships better with far less drama because even confrontation doesn't have to involve conflict.

Poison from the Past

The people that irritate us have a lot in common with poison ivy. Although we don't actually get a rash when we're around them, it just feels like it. It's not commonly known, but whenever anyone becomes exposed to poison ivy for the first time they have no physical reaction. In fact, the vast majority of people have no idea they've even come into contact with the toxic plant. Even so, on the unseen level beneath the skin's surface there is plenty going on. The body absorbs the antigen from the poison ivy, breaks it down, and produces antibodies against it which it stores in the vacuoles (tiny cavities within tissue) for later use. It's only when a person comes into contact with poison ivy a second time that the typical rash, itching, and blisters appear. In order for the unpleasant effects of the secondary exposure to occur, there must have been a primary exposure at some point in time even if a person can't remember it.

Our subconscious works in much the same way. When we get emotionally triggered by another person, it's a similar process as the body having a physical reaction to a biological irritant to which it's been previously exposed. Our anger, irritation, resentment, or jealousy is the emotional blistering or secondary conflict we feel that's actually the reaction from an older, primary emotional conflict of which we're entirely unaware or that we've long forgotten.

Missing the Mark

In medicine, there's an overwhelming tendency to focus on symptoms or effects rather than the cause of illness. With the proliferation of thousands of different drugs today, it's much easier—and more profitable—to write someone a prescription to treat their symptoms rather than taking the time to discover what's actually causing them and eliminate disease at its primary level. In the same way, it's very easy to mistake a person that irritates us and the upset we feel as our primary conflict, especially when we're triggered in a powerful way. We think that if we can get them to come over to our way of thinking or do something we want them to do then all the pain will go away, at least until we're exposed to the next romantic partner, boss, or co-worker who irritates us in the same way. In both medicine and emotions, we tend to focus solely on the secondary conflict, fighting to get what we want in the moment versus discovering what we really need in the long run so nothing actually gets solved or healed.

Owning Our Emotions

Another interesting fact about poison ivy is that after the primary exposure not everyone gets a severe rash and blistering on repeated contact. Some people have no reaction at all. In a similar fashion, not everyone at work is irritated by that jerk in the office to the extent that you are. Why is that?

There's an old saying that goes *you spot it; you got it*. That means you can't have a conscious reaction to something unless there's a corresponding element of it inside of you, too. For example, think back to the last time you bought a new car. In the following months, you suddenly started noticing your car all over the roads driven by other people at stoplights, in parking lots, and on the highway. You were noticing all the different colors and styles whereas only a year ago in your old car, 50 of those cars could drive by you completely unnoticed.

What changed? Was there suddenly more of that kind of car on the road? No. You got one of those cars for yourself and now it was in your consciousness. Because of that, you started seeing it everywhere. In the same way we acknowledge ourselves as the owners of our cars, we have to own all of our emotions and not blame our reactions on other people if we intend to improve our most difficult relationships. At the end of the day, no one can make us feel anything. Present feelings arise from thoughts based on our past experiences.

If you notice your mother-in-law's tendency to be controlling and it upsets you, then her behavior is triggering a deeper issue within you from a previous relationship that has something to do with control, freedom, or independence. This isn't an excuse for anyone's bad behavior but an opportunity to see your reaction to this secondary conflict as a calling to explore your situation a little deeper. Your present upset is an invitation to resolve a primary conflict so that you aren't as triggered in your current relationship and can deal with this person in a calm, conscious manner regardless of how they choose to behave.

Eventually, as you consciously change the way you act and react with this person, they will either change the way they behave toward you or redirect their irritating energy at someone else because you've healed the underlying emotional infectious agent that corresponds with their toxic attitude. You also take back emotional control over your life.

Asking the Right Questions

Whenever you find yourself triggered, the most important and difficult thing to do is to refer inwardly instead of attacking outwardly. It's to ask yourself, *"Regardless of how awful this person is behaving, what does this situation have to say about me?" "How could I have drawn this person or situation into my life?"* Go beyond what you want in the moment and identify the feelings the situation is bringing up for you. *"Why do I feel disrespected?" "When have I felt unloved before?" "How have I or someone else taken me for granted?"*

Through a process known as projection, the subconscious gives us a valuable tool to answer many of these questions. It causes us to project our primary unresolved conflicts outward onto other people just like a movie projector shines an image on a screen where we can see it. The key lies in recognizing that our external or secondary conflict is really an illusion, a trick of the light, and that its primary source is inside of us.

For example, a wife that always criticizes her husband because he never says she's beautiful almost certainly doesn't believe herself that she's beautiful. As such, she projects this subconscious insecurity outward onto her husband for external validation. Perhaps her primary conflict was based in a memory of someone once saying she'd be beautiful, "...if she only lost some weight." Now, even at a healthy weight, she still can't see herself as beautiful. When this primary conflict is resolved, she won't be affected whether her husband does or doesn't comment on her beauty because she'll see her own beauty and be in charge of her own emotions.

Emotional Growth Fuels Advancement

Doing this kind of work isn't just important for emotional and spiritual development. Accomplishing our goals in life is also largely dependent on identifying and resolving the primary emotional conflicts in our lives. Otherwise, our unconscious and uncontrolled reactions and the behaviors that arise from them will hold us back. How many times does someone have to be fired or divorced before they realize, *"Maybe it's not all about everyone else. Maybe it has something to do me."*

If we think about physical life as moving along a horizontal X axis and our spiritual life rising on a vertical Y axis, it's easier to understand how what does or doesn't occur in the emotional realm affects everything in our physical world. It's the cultivation of things like love, courage, trust, authenticity, and self-awareness in our emotional world that fuels our forward momentum into a better life in the physical world and helps us accomplish more of what we want, including the kinds of relationships we'd like to have.

Conflicts and Health Consequences

Success in the physical world includes good health and as I said in an earlier chapter, over time, the stress and negative energy from unresolved primary conflicts, regardless of whether we're conscious of them or not, will take their toll on our bodies. Whenever you're upset on the emotional plane, you can be sure there is a corresponding reaction happing on the physical plane inside your body. At first, these changes are biochemical and go largely unnoticed until they affect us at the cellular level and eventually manifest in physical symptoms. This is why no one gets sick "out of the blue" because chronic conditions build momentum over time, slowly feeding off our stress and anxiety.

I recently saw a patient who was diagnosed with advanced tongue cancer. Her tumor was so large that all the other doctors she'd seen recommended having her entire tongue removed which would have meant never speaking or swallowing again. I soon learned she had a terrible relationship with her ex-husband. He'd been verbally abusive in their marriage during which she felt she had to hold her tongue most of the time. It was near the end of the marriage and in the following years where she developed the habit of literally biting the side of her tongue when dealing with the stress of the situation.

I firmly believe that it was the negative energy from her anger and the belief that she didn't have the right to speak up on her own behalf that was transferred into the tongue through her nervous habit and played a part in her cancer. After working with her to discover the primary injury that caused her to silence herself, I was able to address that issue and help her deal with her ex-husband in a way that served her and improved her experience of that relationship.

After several months of physical treatment and doing this emotional work, her body responded. Her tumor had shrunk to the point where surgeons were finally optimistic that they could remove it without taking the tongue. She would still need physical therapy afterward, but she wouldn't be debilitated.

A Common Journey

Our unresolved primary conflicts can even set our children up for their own disastrous relationships if we don't learn how to parent from a conscious perspective. Since earning my Master of Spiritual Psychology degree, I see many people through my Transformational Intensive and Couples Transformational Intensive self-awareness workshops that experience profound breakthroughs in resolving primary conflicts. The amazing thing is that even though a person may come to me to improve a particular relationship, once they understand this work all their relationships improve, including the one they have with themselves.

When you have to interact with someone who pushes your emotional buttons or becomes defensive, it's important to recognize their divine essence. All this means is that you can see them as another struggling soul trying to work out their own primary conflicts, most of which they're totally unconscious. Just that shift in perspective can be enough to cultivate some compassion and de-escalate the emotional reaction from your side. Keep in mind they're on the same journey of emotional maturity and spiritual development as you. They're just taking a different path.

Perception checking goes a long way toward calming the other person down if things get out of hand. This basically means repeating back to the person what they said to you so they can be reassured you know what's important to them. Most often, all we want in the heat of the moment is to be heard and understood. This is done by saying things like, *"Just so I understand, you..."* or *"It sounds to me like you're saying..."* followed by a short paraphrase of what they've shared.

If you find yourself getting heated, practice self-referral. After the fact, go within and ask the right questions that can lead you to how or why you might be feeling the way that you do and what primary conflicts might be involved in your reactions.

Keep in mind, this kind of work does not mean you must allow yourself to be verbally abused or that you can't speak your mind. It does, however, give you a more positive way of taking control of the situation and yourself. It's the essence of what I call transforming a confrontation into a carefrontation because you can approach it with love for yourself, concern for the other person, and respect for the healing process.

Chapter 10

After the Affair

Saving your marriage from infidelity

Aside from losing a spouse to death, perhaps the most traumatic event a marriage can experience is infidelity. In many respects, infidelity seems to be an insurmountable problem. The faithful spouse finds it impossible to overcome their feelings of betrayal and to trust their partner again. Assuming the cheating spouse wants to save the marriage, he or she can't seem to work through their guilt much less understand why their partner hasn't got over the incident several years later. Both partners can get so caught up in the ensuing emotional drama that neither takes the time, either separately or together, to explore the deeper reason as to why the affair happened in the first place.

In the Internet Age, infidelity has taken on a whole new meaning. With so many social media options, the line between what it means to be faithful or unfaithful to one's spouse is becoming blurred. Some feel chatting with a single co-worker online while texting or trading photos without a spouse's knowledge is unfaithful even though a physical affair has not occurred. Others feel that confiding in someone other than your spouse in a deeply emotional way for support and connection is akin to having an emotional affair.

When it comes to infidelity, you must decide where your boundaries are and what kinds of behavior are unacceptable for you. For the purposes of this discussion, we examine healing a marriage after a physical affair has occurred. Aside from an affair, these steps apply to almost any situation where both parties are willing to work very, very hard to save their relationship through rebuilding trust, communication, and reconnecting. It's not easy, but it's not impossible either.

For the Unfaithful Spouse

Stop the affair immediately

Sever all contact with your lover. This goes way beyond in-person meetings. No phone calls, texts, emails, or contact of any kind is permitted. This eliminates secrecy and is the first step in rebuilding trust with the betrayed partner. Trust is the feeling that one is safe in the relationship. If you work with the person you had the affair with, keep contact businesslike and to an absolute minimum. Share with your spouse every interaction you had with this person *before* he or she has to ask about it. Likewise, you should share any attempts by your former lover to contact you and any chance meetings where you've run into each other. Offer this information in an open and willing manner. You should also plan on looking for a new job immediately to prove that you are serious about total separation from your former lover. This will show you're serious about rebuilding trust and healing your marriage.

If it hasn't happened already, break off contact with your lover over the phone with your spouse present. Let the other person know your spouse is hearing the conversation and that you are under no pressure to break things off. This is your decision to save your marriage and that the call will be your last contact of any kind.

Take responsibility

Blaming your partner for the affair won't heal your marriage. Apologize, and *apologize often* without being prompted. Show sincere remorse and regret for betraying your spouse and vow never to do it again. Ask for forgiveness, realizing that you may not receive it for quite some time. Ask anyway, then ask again. Understand that while you may be sure you'll never stray again your spouse has absolutely no way of being certain of that. Each apology and plea for forgiveness needs to be has heartfelt and genuine as the first even if you're saying it for the one-millionth time. If you're serious about healing your marriage, you'll understand that your spouse needs to hear your apologies many times in many ways before he or she can begin to believe them. Never, ever say to your spouse, "Get over it." If you want him or her to release their pain, then you have to receive it.

Answer all questions honestly and completely

Brutal honesty is key to healing from infidelity. Be ready for your spouse to ask very detailed questions and be equally prepared to answer every one of them. Resist getting frustrated when your spouse asks the same questions repeatedly. This is particularly the case with men who understandably find being cheated on extremely emasculating. A husband may ask about details regarding his wife's sexual encounters with her lover and how those interactions compared with their own. You must be able to handle very uncomfortable conversations and know that withdrawing is not an option.

Many couples, particularly if they are from certain generations, simply don't talk about an affair once it has been discovered. They just keep going through their daily motions. That's not healing; that's avoidance that leads to resentment and further degradation of the marriage over time. Your spouse will ask for exactly what they need in order to heal right down to the finest details. Be ready to supply them as often as needed. Remember, you're rebuilding trust. Don't hold anything back because you're afraid of hurting your spouse. You've already hurt them as much as you possibly can. If you leave out details that emerge later, your spouse will feel newly betrayed.

Practice total transparency

Be willing to offer your spouse all passwords for your cell phone, email, and social media accounts. Don't wait for him or her to have to ask you. Do not erase any old messages from your lover in an attempt to protect your spouse from further hurt. This will only increase fears that you're hiding something.

Be reliable

You have violated your partner's trust at the deepest level. You can start to repair that injury by being trustworthy in all aspects of your relationship. Do you call when you say you will? Do you show up for your spouse where you're supposed to be and on time? If not, do you reach out in advance to give your spouse notice and make other arrangements? Go out of your way to let your spouse know he or she can count on you.

Prepare to be insulted or attacked often

The emotional surges that come with being betrayed may lead your spouse to lash out at you unannounced and unprovoked at times. Don't fire back. Allow your spouse to express his or her pain while reminding them how much you regret the affair, how sorry you are, and how committed you are to healing the relationship. This doesn't mean you have to allow yourself to be verbally abused, but do your best to de-escalate the situation by reassuring your spouse of your love and loyalty. Just don't expect fast or easy forgiveness.

Show empathy

The single best indicator of whether a relationship will survive an affair is the degree to which you are able to show your spouse empathy. To survive the long-term emotional rollercoaster of the situation and not become impatient, irritated or self-righteous, you must be able to put yourself in your spouse's shoes. Professionals often compare the effects of an affair to post traumatic stress disorder (PTSD) that comes with intrusive thoughts and images, racing mind, high anxiety, panic, and confusion.

On average, it takes three to five years to process an affair for the betrayed spouse so they can get to the point where their relationship begins to feel somewhat normal again. Be patient and provide support during this time. Check in with your spouse regularly to ask how they're doing. If they say not so good, just provide reassurance that you'll be there for whatever they need. Let your spouse call the shots in your relationship for the foreseeable future. She doesn't want to go to the football party? Don't bother her about it. Stay home with her while she does gardening in the backyard and find something else to do. Go with the flow for now, and don't press for sex either.

Recognize your feelings

In some cases, the unfaithful spouse can actually feel a sense of loss at ending the affair and disloyalty to their lover for breaking it off. This doesn't mean you love your spouse any less nor are such feelings unusual. Recognize them as normal without adding more guilt to your burden and be sure to discuss them with a counselor.

Infidelity is forever

Trust is far more easily given than it is regained. Rebuilding it is a long-term process. Once broken, however, it will never be the same. That doesn't mean your marriage can't be good and healthy again. It's just that it can never be the same as it was before the affair. After being shattered, a beautiful vase can be repaired to hold water once again, but there will always be visible reminders of the previous damage.

For the Betrayed Spouse

Ask lots of questions

Your mind will be racing and reaching for answers. The more information you have the less likely your mind will be to fill in the blanks with images and scenarios that are even more painful than what actually happened. *How often did you meet? When did you cross the line from friends to lovers? What sexual acts did you share? How many times? Where? How much money did you spend on him or her? Who else knows about your affair?*

Later, your focus may shift to the emotional connection, if any, between your spouse and the lover or how the affair evolved over time. Just keep asking the questions as they come up. Not only will they help you, but they may eventually shine a light on a hidden weakness in your marriage.

Balance your need for information with your rage

Your spouse will be more apt to answer your questions when they feel it won't become a screaming marathon. Yes, it's absolutely necessary to release your rage and your spouse deserves his or her full portion, but try to separate these moments from real factfinding on your part. You might want to consider setting aside specific moments and limited amounts of time to talk with your spouse about the affair. Doing so in intervals gives you time to digest the devastating details in small amounts before moving on to further information. It also helps to keep you from being overwhelmed by everything and prevents the affair from consuming your life.

Focus on your feelings

In discussions with your spouse, be very clear about how his or her behavior made you feel. Was it betrayed, abandoned, inadequate, angry, old, useless, unattractive, or something else? Don't hold back. Give them every chance to validate how their actions harmed you.

Find Support

You can't survive an affair by broadcasting it to everyone. The idea isn't to get everyone on your side or to trash your spouse to all your family and friends. If you want to save your marriage, find one friend who is a great listener and share regularly with them. Destroying your spouse's reputation will only destroy your marriage.

Rebuild your confidence

An affair devastates a person's confidence on every level. Suddenly, you find yourself feeling insecure about your looks, weight, sexual performance, income, and everything else. Do not allow yourself to be consumed by insecurity and the idea that the affair occurred because you're not enough of something. If you don't know your spouse's lover, resist the urge to seek them out or look them up online. That will only incite more pain and comparison. Instead, work to build your own confidence up by changing the way you dress, starting a workout regimen, changing jobs, or pursuing another activity that makes you feel good about yourself.

Building confidence both in and out of the bedroom is essential for your long-term emotional health regardless of whether or not your marriage survives. Erotic recovery is absolutely essential after an affair. It may be a year or more before you can have sex with your spouse again. Don't rush it. When that time comes, pay attention to how he or she makes you feel. Do they make you feel safe? Beautiful? Desirable? Do they build you up both in and outside the bedroom?

Don't forgive quickly or easily

You have a right to your anger and sadness. Be sure it has been fully expressed and a reasonable amount of trust has been reestablished between you and your spouse before you even consider forgiveness. What's forgiven too quickly doesn't stay forgiven. Take as long as you need. You'll know when the time is right.

When you do forgive, let it be genuine. A sure way to doom your marriage is to turn the affair into a life sentence for your spouse. Keep in mind that while you'll never forget the affair it's normal to feel anxiety or have minor trust issues about it even years later. That doesn't mean you haven't forgiven.

Attend therapy

It's highly advised that you both attend therapy separately and together. Friends are wonderful as listeners, but to survive an affair you'll benefit immensely from professional help. Have the courage to honestly evaluate the condition of your marriage before the affair. Infidelity has a way of making previously hidden problems or unexpressed desires of the unfaithful spouse come into view. Be real and honest about your behavior and choices. Did you act in ways that could have been perceived as distant, unkind, or unloving? Sexual and emotional abandonment are common reasons for affairs, but infidelity happens in excellent relationships, as well.

Dig deep and be willing to admit your own faults. In nearly all cases, people don't have affairs because the lover is younger, thinner, richer, or anything else. People have affairs because of the way the other person makes them feel. Pay special attention to how your actions prior to the affair may or may not have made your spouse feel. This isn't to assign blame. There is never an excuse for an affair. This is about how to live a more loving, connected, and fulfilling life together after the affair.

Spend time together

It's important to reconnect as friends first. Go for a picnic or bike ride. Take a Sunday drive together through the country. Continue to live your lives even in spite of the affair and create new experiences and memories together when you're not talking about the affair. You'll have to come together as friends first before you can even contemplate your relationship as spouses again.

Find reasons to stay

If you don't have a big enough reason to make your marriage work, you won't survive the rough times ahead. There is nothing like having a history with someone, and maybe you don't want to start over again with someone new after investing 23 years in a marriage. Maybe you love the fact that there is so much between you and your spouse that doesn't need explaining that life feels free and easy in many ways. Find reasons about your spouse and your life together that you loved before the affair and become committed to saving them. It's not wise to use children as a reason to stay, especially if the marriage is truly irreparable or dangerous. The reason for staying must involve you and your spouse.

Choose to love again

Commit to doing this work long-term because you deserve to love again. You can love each other even in the midst of the pain.

Chapter 11

Conscious Uncoupling

Ending a relationship with integrity and awareness

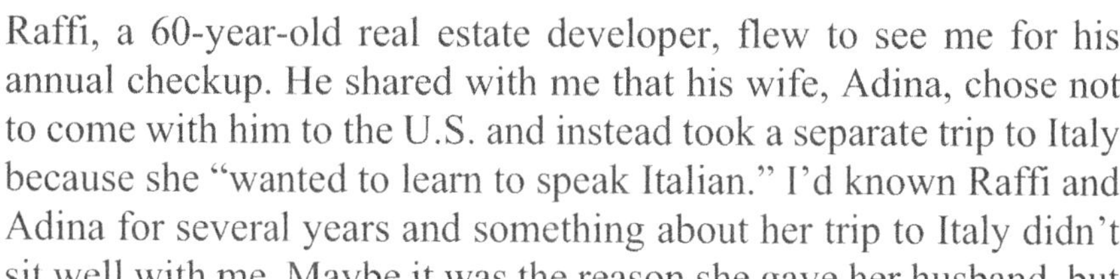

Raffi, a 60-year-old real estate developer, flew to see me for his annual checkup. He shared with me that his wife, Adina, chose not to come with him to the U.S. and instead took a separate trip to Italy because she "wanted to learn to speak Italian." I'd known Raffi and Adina for several years and something about her trip to Italy didn't sit well with me. Maybe it was the reason she gave her husband, but my instinct told me something was amiss.

Three days later, I received a call from Raffi. He had arrived back home to be immediately served with divorce papers from Adina. The majority of his belongings had been gathered up and left in the foyer, a not-so-subtle clue that he was to leave that evening. Looking around his home, he was stunned to see that all the photos of him had already been taken off the walls.

After spending the night in a hotel, he went back to his home the next day to retrieve some additional belongings only to find all the locks had been changed. Calls to his children weren't being returned and, to add insult to injury, all his bank accounts had been frozen.

I knew something about Raffi's background. To me, this was history repeating itself. His mother had left his father virtually overnight when he was a boy. He never saw his father again, and a few years later his father died of a heart attack.

In the coming days, I tried to explain to Raffi the parallels between his past and present situation. Internal healing needed to take place before he too created an even bigger disaster for himself, but he wasn't having any of it. He was completely emotionally saturated in the drama of his material circumstances. I had never seen anyone so consumed with anxiety, rage, depression, and confusion.

I firmly believe that there is a line of trans-generational energy that runs down through families and passes on thought and behavior patterns to us in much the same way our biology passes on our genes. Unresolved emotions from the past traumas of our parents, grandparents, and those before them can be passed down and lead us to unconsciously manifest similar circumstances in our own lives until we recognize the energetic pattern and neutralize it through healing.

When we do so, we not only heal our own lives but break the chain of unknowingly passing negative energetic signatures down to future generations as well. I was praying that after a few days Raffi's shock would subside and I could help him work through the deeper issues of his experience before he created another unintended disaster for himself.

When my phone rang a few weeks later, Raffi's anxiety had continued to escalate. He was throwing up blood and lots of it. It was clear he was hemorrhaging internally and I begged him to go to the emergency room.

Tests would later reveal that his relentless anxiety over his divorce had created a massive bleeding ulcer in his stomach. It was so big that it couldn't be treated orally or through cauterization. He had to be rushed into emergency surgery.

Raffi lost so much blood that his hemoglobin count after surgery was 6.5 g/dL. To put this into perspective, a normal hemoglobin level for a one-year-old baby is 11 g/dL while an adult man should range between 14 and 17 g/dL. Raffi would eventually lose 45 lbs. and spend weeks recovering in intensive care from an experience that nearly cost him his life just like his father.

Sometimes, hitting rock bottom is the greatest gift a person can receive. In Raffi's case, that's exactly what happened. After leaving the hospital and regaining some of his strength, we began to work together on his emotional healing. I can't express what a monumental challenge this was for a man whose wife was leaving him because, among other reasons, he was emotionally unavailable. Even though none of the circumstances surrounding his divorce had changed, he chose to step out in faith and work on his inner emotional world, believing that somehow it would positively impact his outer world.

Two weeks before Raffi's divorce hearing, Adina responded to a text he had sent her agreeing to have lunch with him. This was the first direct contact they'd had with each other in months. Over the course of the conversation, they were both brought to tears at the ending of their 25 years together. It was quite possibly the most candid and emotionally open they had ever been with each other during their entire marriage. While Adina still felt she needed to move on, she agreed to arbitration instead of going through with what would have been a long, protracted public battle in the courts.

Today Raffi has a healthy relationship with all of his children and makes it a priority to spend time with them and his grandchildren. While still a man of international business, he's learned that the most important business from which he'll profit the most is right at home.

Until Death Do Us Part

Divorce is a difficult decision and traumatic experience for everyone involved, but does it have to be so antagonistic? Currently, 43% of all first marriages end in divorce.[1] That's down from 50% in 2000. Even so, many people are concerned about the divorce rate and see it as a problem that needs to be fixed, but what if divorce isn't really a problem?

What if, when the whole concept of marriage and divorce is reexamined, there's actually something far more powerful and positive at play? What if divorce is just a symptom of something deeper that needs our attention? The high divorce rate might actually be a calling to learn a new way of being in relationships.

During the upper Paleolithic period of human history (roughly 50,000 BC to 10,000 BC) the average human life expectancy at birth was 33.[2] By 1900, U.S. life expectancy had risen to 46 for men and 48 for women. Today it's 76 and 80 respectively.[3] During the 52,000 years between our Paleolithic ancestors and the dawn of the 20th century, life expectancy rose just 15 years. In the last 124 years, it increased 30 years for men and 32 years for women.

What does this have to do with divorce rates? For the vast majority of history, humans lived relatively short lives. They weren't in relationships with the same person for 30 to 50 years. Modern society adheres to the concept that marriage should be lifelong, but when we are living three lifetimes compared to early humans, perhaps we need to redefine the construct. Social research suggests that because we are living so long, most people will have two or three significant long-term relationships in their lifetime.

With regard to relationship longevity, as divorce rates indicate, human beings haven't been able to fully adapt to our skyrocketing life expectancy. This isn't to suggest there aren't couples who remain happily married for 30, 40, or 50 years. We all hope that we're one of them. Everyone enters into marriage with the good intention to go all the way. Accomplishing this requires occasionally redefining who we are separately within the relationship and discovering new ways of being together as we change and grow.

It's also important to remember that just because someone is still married doesn't mean they're happy or that the relationship is fulfilling. To that end, living happily ever after for the length of a 21st century lifetime should not be the yardstick by which we define a successful intimate relationship. This is an important consideration as we reform the concept of divorce.

The Honeymoon Ends

Nearly everyone comes into a new marriage idealizing their partner. Everything is perfect in their minds because they've misidentified what marriage is really about. As far as they're concerned, they've found the love of their life, the person who understands them completely. Yes, there will be hiccups along the way but, by and large, there's no more learning left to do. They'll both be the same people 10 or 20 years from now as they are today.

When we idealize our partners, things initially go very well as we subconsciously project our own positive qualities as well as the qualities we wish we had onto them. This positive projection happens during the honeymoon phase of the relationship where both partners can do no wrong in each other's eyes.

Sooner or later the honeymoon ends and reality sets in—and with it the negative projection of the "witch" begins. We stop projecting positive things onto our partner and begin to project our negative issues instead. This creates a boomerang effect. These negative issues always come right back to us, triggering our unconscious and long-buried negative hurts, betrayals, and traumas.

For most of us, these unresolved issues can be traced back to our first intensely emotional relationship, the one we had with our parents. Because most of these old wounds are unconscious to us as adults, we're subconsciously driven to resolve them which is why many people end up with partners that are very similar in key ways to their mother or father. As such, our partner is a setup for the "witch."

If we're not in tune with this type of dynamic within our relationship, all we end up seeing is the repeated mistrust, abandonment, or other issue that has followed us through all our previous relationships. We never see that it's the signal to heal the emotional wound that's connected to it. Instead, we choose to blame the other person.

Because we believe so strongly in the "until death do us part" concept, we see the demise of our marriage as a failure, bringing with it shame, guilt, or regret. Since most of us don't want to face what we see as a personal failure, we retreat into resentment and anger. As we resort to attacking each other, we fail to see the emotional armor we have amassed over the years to defend ourselves is our real problem.

While a full body shield may offer a level of self-protection, it's also a form of self-imprisonment that locks us inside a life that repeats the same mistakes over and over again. This includes attracting the same kind of partners to push the same emotional buttons for us until we recognize the deeper purpose of such a relationship.

Intimacy & Insects

To understand what life is really like living with an external shield, we have to examine the experts. Beetles, grasshoppers, and all other insects have an exoskeleton. The structure that protects and supports their body is on the outside. Not only are they stuck in a rigid form that provides no flexibility, they are also at the mercy of their environment. If they find themselves under the heel of a shoe, it's all over. That's not the only downside. Their exoskeletons can calcify, leading to more rigidity.

Vertebrates like dogs, horses, and humans have an endoskeleton. Our support structure is on the inside of our bodies, giving us exceptional flexibility and mobility to adapt and change under a wide range of circumstances. The price for this gift is vulnerability because our soft outside is completely exposed to hurt and harm every day.

Life is a spiritual exercise in evolving from an exoskeleton for support and survival to an endoskeleton. When we get our emotional support and wellbeing from outside ourselves, our moods are at the mercy of our environment since we can't control what another person does. Anything someone says or does can set us off and ruin our day. If our intimate partner doesn't behave the way we think they should, everything is perceived as a personal attack and an attempt to upset us. Up goes our armor and it's all-out war.

With an internal support structure, we can stand strong because our stability doesn't depend on anything outside ourselves. We can be vulnerable and pay attention to what's happening around us, knowing that whatever comes, we have the flexibility to adapt to the situation. There's a reason we call cowards spineless. It takes great courage to drop your armor, expose your soft inside, and come to terms with the reality of what's happening around you.

It's a powerful thing to then realize that you can survive it. When we examine our intimate relationships from this perspective, we realize that they aren't for finding static, lifelong bliss like we see in the movies. They're for helping us develop a psycho-spiritual spine, a divine endoskeleton made from conscious self-awareness so that we can evolve into a better life without recreating the same problems for ourselves again and again.

When we learn to find our emotional and spiritual support from inside ourselves, nothing that changes our external environment or relationships can unsettle us. Situations we once viewed as problems will be seen as opportunities to reflect inwardly and determine what each one is trying to reveal to us about ourselves. Problems are transmuted into opportunities for growth.

Millions of years ago insects were enormous. A dragonfly's wings were three feet across. So why didn't they end up being the dominant species on earth? Russian philosopher Peter Ouspensky came to the conclusion that the creation of insects was a failed attempt by nature to evolve a higher form of consciousness. Since they lacked flexibility, which is what evolution is all about, they couldn't adapt to changing conditions like humans can.

The lives of people who imprison themselves in an exoskeleton of anger usually don't evolve the way they would like. Being trapped inside negative energy like resentment keeps people from moving forward in life because they can only focus on the past. Even worse, over time these powerful emotions often turn into disease in the body.

Conscious Uncoupling

To change our concept of divorce, we need to release the belief structure we have around marriage that creates rigidity in our thought process. The belief structure is the all-or-nothing idea that when we marry it's for life. The truth is the only thing any of us have is today. Beyond that there are no guarantees. The idea of being married to one person for life, especially without some level of awareness of our unresolved emotional issues, is too much pressure for anyone.

In fact, it would be interesting to see how much easier couples might commit to each other by thinking of their relationship in terms of daily renewal instead of a lifetime investment. This is probably the reason why so many people say their long-term relationships changed overnight once they got married. While the people didn't change, their expectations did. It's odd that most of us assume that everything in a relationship will stay the same based on a single promise made during a wedding ceremony and that somehow no further work is required for the marriage to remain intact.

If we can recognize that partners in our intimate relationships aren't the witches we've come to think of them as but teachers who help us evolve our internal spiritual support structure, we can avoid the drama of divorce and experience what's known as a *conscious uncoupling*.

The idea of uncoupling as an alternative to a nasty divorce has been around since the 1970s. In 1990, author Diane Vaughan further defined the concept while psychotherapist Katherine Woodward Thomas would popularize it a few years later. In these previous theories, uncoupling is rooted in how to part amicably, keeping mutual respect as part of the process and remembering the needs of any children involved.[4]

While these are admirable and necessary steps for a conscious uncoupling, self-reflection must be the foundation of the process if we are to avoid repeating the same problems in the next relationship. The idea of conscious uncoupling is to gain enough self-awareness that we no longer have to go through the same drama again because we've now found ourselves in a fulfilling and sustainable long-term relationship.

For our purposes here, conscious uncoupling is the ability to understand that every irritation and argument within a relationship is a signal to look inside ourselves and identify an unresolved emotional issue that needs healing. Because present events always trigger pain from a past event, it's never the current situation that needs fixing. The present hurt is just the echo of an older emotional injury. If we can remain conscious of this during our uncoupling, we will understand that how we relate to ourselves internally as we go through an experience is the real issue, not the external details of what's happening.

From this perspective, there are no bad guys just two people playing teacher and student respectively. When we understand that both are actually partners in each other's spiritual progress, animosity dissolves much more quickly and a new paradigm for conscious uncoupling emerges to replace the traditional contentious divorce.

It's only under these circumstances that loving co-parenting can happen. Conscious uncoupling prevents families from being broken by divorce and creates expanded families that continue to function in a healthy way outside of traditional marriage. Children are imitators by nature, and as parents we teach what we *are*. If we are to raise a more conscious and civilized generation, we must model this behavior through the choices we make during the good and bad times in our relationships.

Wholeness in Separation

It seems contradictory to say that a marriage coming apart is the cause of something else coming together, but it's true. Conscious uncoupling brings wholeness to the spirits of both people who choose to recognize each other as their teacher. If they do, the gift they receive from their time together will neutralize their negative internal issues that were the real cause of their pain in the relationship.

This dynamic is in play in all of our personal relationships, not just the intimate ones. If we can allow ourselves this gift, our exoskeleton of protection and imprisonment will fall away and offer us the opportunity to begin constructing an endoskeleton, an internal support structure built on self-love, self-acceptance, and self-forgiveness.

This process allows us to begin projecting something different into the world because we have regained a missing part of our heart. Such an addition to our psychic infrastructure creates a wholeness that supports our own growth and ability to co-parent consciously.

Coming Together

The misunderstandings involved in divorce also have much to do with the lack of intercourse between our own internal masculine and feminine energies. Choosing to hide within an exoskeleton and remain in attack mode requires a great imbalance of masculine energy. Feminine energy is the source of peacemaking, nurturing, and healing.

Regardless of whether you're a man or woman, cultivating your feminine energy during this time is beneficial to the success of conscious uncoupling. When our masculine and feminine energies reach equilibrium once more, we can emerge from our old relationship and consciously attract a partner who reflects our new world, not the old one.

Naturally, divorce is much easier if both parties choose to have a conscious uncoupling. Even so, your experience and personal growth aren't conditional on whether or not your spouse chooses to participate. You can still receive the lessons he or she has to give you by resisting being baited into dramatic arguments and standing firm in your internal support system. By choosing to handle your uncoupling in a conscious way regardless of how your spouse might be behaving, you'll see that although it looks like everything is coming apart, it's actually coming back together.

Chapter 12

The Elusive Orgasm

Why many women can't climax

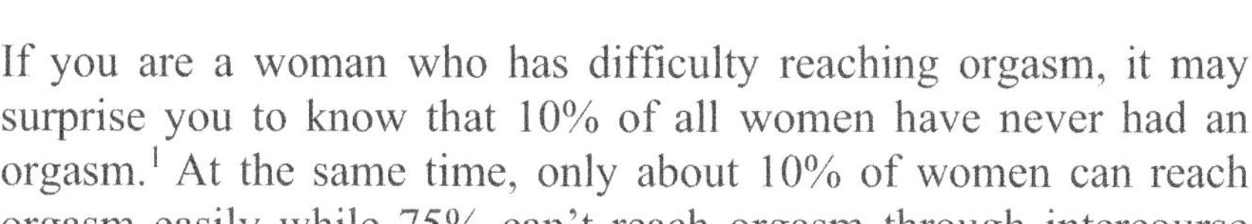

If you are a woman who has difficulty reaching orgasm, it may surprise you to know that 10% of all women have never had an orgasm.[1] At the same time, only about 10% of women can reach orgasm easily while 75% can't reach orgasm through intercourse alone without the aid of sex toys or oral/manual masturbation.[2] [3] Overall, women only reach orgasm about 50% to 70% of the time.[4]

Unfortunately, misunderstanding the female orgasm can leave women questioning whether they're "normal" and their partners feeling inadequate when their efforts to satisfy them fail. The good news is, in most cases, there is nothing wrong with either partner because the sexual response in women is more complex than it is for men. When it's better understood, sex becomes more satisfying and consistent for both partners. Much of it has to do with how the female body is constructed.

What's normal?

The closer a woman's clitoris is to her vaginal opening, the more likely she is to be able to climax from intercourse alone. The ideal clitoris to vagina measurement or C-V distance is 2.5cm or about one inch. Any further separation will prevent the clitoris from receiving adequate stimulation during penetration. Many women needlessly worry because they've never had an orgasm through intercourse but can easily reach one through masturbation. Of course, this is normal. Husbands and boyfriends should be educated about C-V distance so there's no pressure that a woman's orgasm has to come from the penis alone because it very rarely does.

At the same time, professor of biology at Indiana University Elisabeth Lloyd provides a credible theory as to why women don't consistently reach orgasm from every sexual encounter and almost never do from intercourse in her book, *The Case of the Female Orgasm*. In contrast to women, 98% of men say they always reach orgasm during sex.[5]

According to Lloyd, the male orgasm is directly connected to ejaculation and therefore essential to continuing the human species. As such, the consistent male orgasm has been highly selected by evolution. Because the female orgasm isn't central to conception, women overwhelmingly don't orgasm during intercourse and sometimes may not reach climax at all. This is evidenced by the fact that a woman's ability to orgasm has no effect on her fertility. In much the same way, nipples are highly sensitive in women as opposed to men because they are also crucial to nourishing the next generation and continuing human life on earth.[6]

With this in mind, rest assured that if it takes you as a woman or your female partner a bit of time to work up to an orgasm, have never had an orgasm from intercourse, or don't make it over the top once in a while then congratulations; you're normal. The women we're focusing on here are those who cannot have an orgasm under any circumstances.

Abuse & Awareness

Anorgasmia, sometimes called female orgasmic disorder (FOD), is the medical term used when a woman cannot reach orgasm and is classified in two ways. Primary anorgasmia occurs when a woman has never experienced an orgasm while secondary anorgasmia relates to women who have experienced orgasm but never again after a certain time in their lives.

Because all women possess the proper anatomy to have an orgasm, there is no reason why those suffering from anorgasmia can't eventually achieve one with relative consistency. First it requires understanding whether the cause of the condition is either physical or psychological and then moving forward with much patience and self-love to do the necessary healing work.

Many women discover that their anorgasmia is connected to some form of emotional, physical, or sexual abuse from their past. Sex may be seen as dangerous causing women to hold back. They may feel it's wrong to enjoy sex or suffer from low self-esteem. Issues with negative body image may also come into play as well as religious and social taboos. All these factors contribute to a woman's inability to remain present during sex, causing her to be preoccupied with sudden feelings of fear, guilt, shame, anger and isolation. It's important to remember that for women who have never experienced orgasm memories of abuse may be subconscious and just beyond their immediate awareness. Women affected by these situations often report experiencing the build-up of sexual tension and then hitting a wall. In these cases, psychotherapy is absolutely essential as is a loving and patient partner. With courage and the right support, many women have overcome their past and achieved the joy of orgasm.

Lack of Intimacy

Touch is important for building the momentum during sex, especially for women, but it has to be the right kind of touch. Most couples say they already touch, hug, and kiss during sex. The question is whether intimacy is involved. Is the touch loving? How long does it last? Is there real, extended eye contact?

How a woman receives and perceives touch makes a great deal of difference as to whether her body is primed for orgasm or not. This isn't to imply that a man is solely responsible for a woman's orgasm, but touch is where every sexual encounter begins. Touch is a powerful form of communication that resonates in every cell of the body and needs no words to make its message known. When a woman feels loved, safe, adored, and even worshipped by the kind of touch she's experiencing, her mind will quiet while the body relaxes and opens into a receptive state that's primed for pleasure.

As we get older and hormone levels start to change, intimate touch becomes an invaluable tool to help us build up to an orgasm that many of us used to achieve in only minutes when we were in our

20's. A University of Chicago study found that women in their 50s and upwards were nearly three times less likely to achieve orgasm when there was little or no intimate touching involved.[7]

Another study found that the optimal amount of time for sexual intercourse was between three and 13 minutes with the average being 7.3.[8] Sadly, this amount of time accounts for the *entire* sexual encounter for some people, not just penetration. During the rest of the time you might want to consider slow or prolonged kissing, spooning, touching the face while keeping eye contact, kissing the forehead, kissing down the length of the arms, legs or torso, laying your head on your partner's chest to hear their heartbeat, or playing with their hair.

Building intimacy in this way is essential to a woman's orgasm. This means taking time and slowing things down, sometimes way down. Letting go of goal-oriented sex where orgasm is the prize greatly reduces sexual expectations and stress and allows the body to progress at its own pace. The reward will be a deepening of your relationship and the opportunity to have experiences that are, in many ways, even more satisfying and longer lasting than a fleeting orgasm.

Relaxation vs. Tension

Orgasm is somewhat of a paradox because as the body approaches climax, it requires the perfect balance between relaxation and tension. How can we be relaxed and tense at the same time? In this case, the body must be in a state of tension while the mind is relaxed or silent. Because the male orgasm is highly selected for sex by evolution and the male thought process is generally linear in nature, it's not very difficult for a man to get his mind into the orgasm zone during sex. Odds are very good that in the heat of the moment, he's not thinking about that business proposal he has to present at the end of the week. Women, however, can have a bigger challenge keeping their mind in the moment.

To minimize distractions, give yourself enough time to have longer, more intimate sex. No more quickies. The time to have sex isn't 30 minutes before you have to leave the house for an appointment. Make sure the kids are taken care of so you don't have to think about them. Even holding back during sex because you're afraid the noise will wake them up is enough distraction to prevent orgasm.

Meditation can be helpful in learning to quiet the mind as is visualizing an abstract concept like white light. If religious or sexual taboos are a distraction, counseling is essential. Regularly introducing new positions, toys, and so on can be a good way to keep your mind in the moment and stop it from zoning out because sex has become routine.

As the mind relaxes, the body needs to become tense. For women, this means the buttocks, thighs, and pelvic floor muscles, the ones you use to stop the flow of urine. Consciously tensing these muscles during oral or manual masturbation and penetration helps increase physical tension. This causes additional blood to engorge the genitals, increasing sensitivity and assisting the body in building to orgasm.

A condition known as pelvic floor prolapse is a loosening of these muscles that support the pelvic organs and can be caused by pregnancy, childbirth, straining from constipation, chronic coughing, or aging. If you leak a few drops of urine when you sneeze, laugh, or cough, this might be an issue for you.

Kegel exercises help tone the pelvic floor muscles and are easy to do. Tense the muscles you use to stop urine flow and hold the contraction for five seconds. Then release for five seconds. Repeat the exercise for a set of 10. Try to get three sets in during the day. You'll want to work your way up to contracting for 10 seconds and releasing for 10. Since this is an internal exercise, there should be no movement of the abdominals or any other visible muscles.

Medications & Surgery

Drugs for depression, anxiety, regulating blood pressure, and sedatives all delay or impede orgasm by preventing the muscles around the vagina and clitoris from becoming adequately engorged with blood which is necessary for sexual pleasure. Consult your physician as to the possibility of reducing your prescription or taking a trial period off the medication to see how your body responds.

Sometimes switching to different medication can make a

difference. Some of the drug companies are now promoting brands they claim come with minimal or no sexual side effects. A clitoris vacuum pump draws extra blood into the clitoris. Used in conjunction with a medication change, it can provide added support.

Significant scarring from injuries or surgeries often blocks one or more of the energetic pathways in the body called meridians. The result is a condition known as reverse polarity. When energy travels down a meridian and hits scar tissue, it either pools and stagnates in this area or ricochets off this roadblock and flows down another meridian where it doesn't belong. In either case, it can create physical problems in the vicinity of the scar or in remote areas of the body. For many women who used to have orgasms but can no longer achieve them, the culprit is often a scar from a C-section birth.

A procedure known as integrative neural therapy injects procaine into the scar tissue. This generates a release of some of the rigidity and stagnant energy. Homeopathic agents are added to accelerate the release and reopen the pathway. We will deal more thoroughly with what to do about scar tissue in the next chapter. The results are often immediate and dramatic. Many women have had sexual pleasure restored to their lives through this method, never suspecting that their C-section scar could have anything to do with the fact that they lost the ability to orgasm shortly after giving birth. The procedure has also been effective in alleviating painful intercourse after a C-section. Interestingly, the Japanese use a vertical incision for C-sections to avoid disrupting the energy meridians of the body.

Hormonal Imbalance

Testosterone is the hormone of desire in women, not estrogen. Although women only need a small amount of testosterone for sexual health, the slightest imbalance is enough to create a big problem such as lack of libido or inability to orgasm. If a larger chronic disease process isn't an issue, hormone levels should be checked by a physician. Bio-identical testosterone is available in a number of different applications. Testosterone creams are available that may be applied directly to the clitoris to heighten sensitivity.

Letting the Body Lead

Understanding the causes of anorgasmia is essential to ending the false assumptions that surround it. Inability to orgasm doesn't mean something is wrong with a relationship or that either partner is inadequate. The best treatment for anorgasmia is to be in a deeply loving, intimate, and patient relationship. This enables both partners to communicate with each other about what works and what doesn't while trying lots of new things.

Healing from anorgasmia can also be achieved outside of a relationship through self-stimulation and, in some ways, may be preferable because there's no perceived pressure to perform. In either case, it's important to remember that every woman is different and orgasm isn't always an earth-shattering experience.

Let go of all your expectations about orgasm and the exaggerated way you've seen it portrayed on TV and in films. That's not reality. The journey to orgasm is a beautiful and very personal one. Just let go, and let your body reveal what orgasm is for *you*.

Chapter 13

The Infertility Illusion

A tilted uterus can prevent conception

After more than a year of trying to conceive naturally without success, Kathy and her husband were frustrated. When a test on her husband's sperm count came back normal, they decided to try multiple rounds of *in vitro* fertilization (IVF). In the process, they spent tens of thousands of dollars only to experience a miscarriage with every attempt.

When she came to me, I asked Kathy about previous injuries for which she had been treated. It turned out that years earlier she had been a cheerleader in college. In a hard fall one day in practice she broke her tailbone. Her previous doctors had assured her that a broken tailbone wouldn't affect her ability to become pregnant.

Examining her, I discovered that she had a tilted uterus. Regardless of what her previous doctors had told her, I corrected the tilted uterus. Just weeks after the treatment, Kathy conceived naturally.

Obvious Answers

There's an old adage that says, "When you hear hoofbeats, look for horses not zebras." In other words, when there are signs of a problem, look for the simplest, most logical explanation. Don't go off on an exotic tangent looking for some complicated far-fetched reason, scaring and stressing yourself out in the process.

Having a child might just be the greatest joy in life for most couples, especially for women. The yearning many women experience to become a mother runs so deep that it's interwoven with their feminine identity and purpose on earth as a human being. More than a desire, it's a primal drive. Men are born with an equally intense compulsion to seek women out and meet that need. Somewhere at the center of our being, most men and women unconsciously understand that carrying on the human species is one of our greatest honors and responsibilities in life. When a couple experiences fertility problems and cannot accomplish this primal purpose, men and women tend to react differently.

If the male is infertile, he tends to struggle with masculinity issues and loses his sense of self. Because women are responsible for 99% percent of the procreation process, childbirth is more intensely integrated into a woman's consciousness. If she happens to be the infertile partner, her pain goes beyond losing her sense of self. She often loses her reason for being. Deep-seated feelings of having no use in the world are common among women who are told they are infertile.

It seems that the women who are struggling to get pregnant are younger every year. It's common now to see women in their 20s and early 30s utilizing assisted reproductive technology (ART). It might be surprising to hear that the simplest reason an otherwise healthy woman cannot become pregnant has nothing to do with her fertility and everything to do with her physical structure, as was the case with Kathy. After being told they have impaired fertility, most women feel that ART is their only option.

Costs of Conception

According to the Centers for Disease Control and Prevention (CDC), a woman is considered infertile if there is no conception after 12 months of unprotected sex with her male partner. Women with multiple miscarriages who have never carried a baby to term are also considered infertile. Among women of child-bearing age between 15 and 49 in the United States, 13.4% are said to have impaired fertility.[1]

As if the emotional rollercoaster of fertility struggles wasn't enough, couples facing fertility challenges are left with few options except ART and the exorbitant costs that come with it. After an initial examination, blood tests, and workup costing about $5,000, the choices include everything from intrauterine insemination from about $1,500 per trial to IVF which starts at around $12,000 per trial. This doesn't include required medications that run between $3,000 and $7,000. While most insurance companies will pay for tests to determine fertility status, they usually won't cover ART services.

Kathy had one of the more common reasons for infertility, a tilted uterus. Because most physicians and patients are entirely unaware that such a condition can exist, couples often end up financially spent and emotionally drained after years of unsuccessful ART attempts. When a uterus is tilted, even the chances of conceiving through IVF are virtually zero.

A Hard Landing

Most women don't realize that when they fall they can land in such a way where the impact creates a misalignment of the uterus. This can occur at a young age and go completely unnoticed because there is often no serious or lasting pain related to the event. For young girls, this can often happen during activities like gymnastics, figure skating, cheerleading, or in any activity where there is a great potential to land heavily on one's bottom.

These incidents are quickly forgotten. As women move forward to start their families, it doesn't occur to them to connect their inability to conceive with these innocuous incidents decades earlier. From every physiological perspective, hormonal and otherwise, these women are quite fertile and completely capable of conceiving a child, but a tilted uterus will never allow that process to take place.

This kind of invisible injury can happen at any point in a woman's life. I recently treated an actress who took a hard landing while filming a stunt on a movie set. After struggling to get pregnant for nearly a year, she came to my office where we discovered her coccyx was completely jammed up, creating a tilt in her uterus. Like most women, she was completely unaware of this condition.

The good news is that in many cases a tilted uterus can be corrected in a painless procedure that greatly improves the chances of conception, saving couples a small fortune and years of heartbreak. If you or a woman you know are struggling with conceiving or maintaining a pregnancy, the first place to look is the uterus. This is the environment where the fertilized egg or zygote needs to attach itself and grow.

Force of Gravity

Assuming the father is fertile and the mother is in good health, any fertilized egg or zygote will be viable. When a zygote fails to result in a birth, suspicion needs to be shifted to the zygote's environment. Until the uterus is properly examined, all attempts at assisted reproductive technology will be wasted time and money. It's highly unlikely an embryo will be able to attach itself and grow in a tilted uterus regardless of the fertility method used.

The uterus rises from the cervix and folds forward to partially rest on the bladder. With the uterus in this position, a fertilized egg can easily travel and come to rest on the inner wall of the flat portion overlaying the bladder. This "shelf" provides a stable base for it to firmly attach and grow. This location also protects the fertilized egg from being disturbed by anything else that might be introduced into the vaginal canal.

Due to a number of reasons, the uterus can end up curving backward at the cervix toward the pelvis. Most physicians refer to this condition as a retroverted or tilted uterus. The severity of the tilt is measured as either first, second, or third degree. In rare cases known as a retroflexed uterus, the tilted uterus can actually fold backward onto itself. This puts pressure on the rectum, creating problems with elimination.

The tilted uterus will either be in a perfectly vertical position behind the bladder or leaning backwards at an angle. When this happens, it's difficult for the fertilized egg to find a proper place to come to rest, attach, and grow. With the uterus now creating a straight channel downward toward the vaginal opening, it's common for the fertilized egg to lose its grip and slide right out of the body.

As it does with the majority of sperm cells, gravity plays a prominent role. In its normal position folded over the bladder, the uterus is like a cul-de-sac with a soft bend in the road and a pocket at the end where the fertilized egg can sit. The tilted uterus is like a vertical, straight, one-way street where the fertilized egg has to hang on for dear life, fighting the forces of gravity where all the traffic moves in one direction, down and out.

Most women with a tilted uterus don't experience pain or any symptoms at all. Others can have rare symptoms that include vaginal pain or lower back pain during sexual intercourse, menstrual pain, trouble inserting tampons, urinary tract infections, and mild incontinence.

Maladies & Misalignment

Sometimes a prior pregnancy can overstretch the ligaments holding the uterus in place, leaving it unable to maintain its natural position so that it falls backward. Scarring from adhesions due to endometriosis or fibroids often pulls the uterus backward and holds it there. When left untreated, sexually transmitted diseases like chlamydia and gonorrhea lead to pelvic inflammatory disease and can cause scarring that results in similar effects to endometriosis. Any scarring from a history of pelvic surgery can also be a cause.

If none of these conditions exist and yet the uterus is still tilted, most doctors will insist that the condition is genetic. Based on the patients I've seen, I have to disagree. Any internal scarring in the pelvic region as a result of injury can cause the uterus to be misaligned. As we saw with Kathy, this happens most in female athletes involved in sports that have a high risk of repeatedly landing on their buttocks. Although seemingly harmless, the repeated impact from these falls often forces the pelvic floor upward into an unnatural position, throwing the uterus out of alignment.

Incomplete Interventions

Once a tilted uterus is diagnosed through a pelvic exam, patients may be prescribed various exercises like knee-chest lifts, pelvic contractions, and Kegels to strengthen ligaments and realign the uterus. Success with exercises is mostly limited and temporary. If scarring is an issue, exercises won't work at all.

Another option is the pessary device, a plastic or silicone application that can be inserted into the vagina to prop the uterus into a better position, but the effect is temporary. When the device is left in long-term, it has been associated with infection.

The only permanent solution that conventional medicine offers for a tilted uterus is surgical. A uterine suspension can be performed to realign the uterus. More recently a laparoscopic version of the same procedure known as a uterine uplift has become available.

Integrative Options

Integrative medicine offers a non-surgical intervention to realign the uterus that is effective in the vast majority of cases. Treatment involves having the patient lie face down on the examining table. Because the uterus is tilted toward the back of the body, the physician must enter through the rectum to perform a number of osteopathic manipulations in order to guide it back into place.

Initially, the procedure involves releasing tension in the pelvic floor. This allows it to relax and move back into its original position, creating more vertical space in which the manipulations can take place. During this phase of the treatment, patients sometimes describe a mild queasy sensation in the pit of their stomach as if they were going over a small rollercoaster hill. Since the work is being done in the vicinity of the bladder, others might experience a phantom urge to urinate.

The second half of the treatment involves a release and rebalancing of the buildup of energy that has been stagnating in and around the reproductive organs. If scarring is present, procaine and homeopathic injections are administered into the nerve plexus to release the rigidity of the tissue, increase its flexibility, and improve its ability to conduct energy. As we discussed earlier, scars anywhere in the body create blockages that cause the body's electrical energy to stagnate in those areas. In order to become pregnant, a woman's body needs to be able to accept the energy she's receiving from her male partner and her own egg. This can't happen if she's energetically saturated because of misalignment or scarring in the area of the uterus.

If energy isn't freely moving, cells can't communicate to operate properly. Electrically speaking, by releasing the pelvic floor and the rigidity of the scar tissue, it's similar to creating an electrical short or override of the system sort of like rebooting a computer. The body's electrical system goes to zero and then immediately realigns with energy flowing freely down all the proper channels, including through the pelvic region.

With no more energy bound up in this area, patients often experience a new sense of wellbeing not realizing that this internal physical tension kept them in a mild state of fight-or-flight that they once thought was their normal state of being. Sometimes the physical release of tension can trigger a simultaneous release of subconscious emotions long forgotten and left over from the original injury.

The entire procedure to correct a tilted uterus takes between 30 and 90 minutes depending on each patient's condition. For cases without scarring or only mild scarring, success rates are high. Depending on the severity of the tilt, scarring, and other issues, more than one session may be necessary. In rare cases where scarring is excessive, surgery may be the best option.

Heavy Metals & Medicines

While the corrective procedure for a tilted uterus is extremely effective, it's important to be aware of several other health and lifestyle issues that can help or harm your fertility regardless of the treatment you choose. Heavy metals like thallium are everywhere and some of the biggest culprits in decreasing fertility. Thallium is used in cell phones, computer equipment, and other technology that requires lithium batteries. Experts worldwide have been urging strict international regulation on its usage.[2] Women undergoing IVF must take care to avoid environmental thallium exposure which can lead to "embryonic arrest" and failure.[3] Heavy metal exposure through various means like eating foods grown in contaminated soil is also largely responsible for the decrease in male fertility.[4]

Dental health is often a mirror for overall physical health. Be sure you don't have any amalgam metal fillings in your teeth. Mercury can leech out from them into the rest of the body, causing all sorts of cognitive and neurological problems as well as contributing to infertility.

Periodontal or gum disease can also contribute to infertility. Inflamed gums and the associated bacteria generate the production of prostaglandin, the hormone that tells the female body it's time to start contractions.[5] This false signal can be the hidden culprit behind miscarriages.

Certain medications can often reduce fertility even though it's not listed as one of the product's side effects. I had a new patient who was devastated when he was diagnosed as infertile. It just so happened that he was taking a medication known as Colchicine for gout. He had no idea that his medication greatly reduced the production of sperm. The active ingredient in Colchicine is what scientists use to sterilize regular watermelon plants to create seedless watermelons. When I took this patient off the medication and substituted it with two natural alternatives and 100% organic cherry juice, his fertility returned to normal and his gout disappeared.

Learning to Let Go

Everything we desire in life has a corresponding state of consciousness that is required to manifest it. Fertility is also a state of consciousness. Before the physical act of trying to conceive even begins, it's important for both partners, but especially women, to begin to move themselves into a state of being that supports fertility.

For women in particular, this requires getting out of the *doing* frame of mind and settling into *being*. It can be tough to slow down and just enjoy a quiet moment, but every chance a woman has to get back into her body and out of her head allows her to settle into her feminine energy more. The body will respond to this emotional shift. Do your best to find things you love about your body because your relationship with your body is your relationship to your feminine energy. Become more in touch physically with the earth. Spend more time in nature. Let Mother Earth infuse you with her fertile energy. If you're constantly overscheduled and running around triggering your stress response, your body is not primed for pregnancy. In fight-or-flight mode, the body thinks an emergency is happening, and that's *not* the time to get pregnant.

Life is a recurring test in how to surrender. One of the key aspects of manifestation is detachment, which means reaching the place of being okay if you don't get what you want. It's the state of consciousness known as negative capability which involves being okay with things *not* being okay and moving forward to accept whatever comes. It's in that place of mental neutrality that magical things happen.

Sometime after my wife and I started dating, I told her that there was a real possibility I might not be able to father a child because of my diagnosis of testicular cancer several years earlier. This revelation caused her to have to unexpectedly deal with the pain I discussed earlier that she might never be a mother. We set our intention to have a family and lived each day in a state of surrender to whatever would be. The result of that choice was two beautiful children.

Fertility is as much a state of mind as it is lifestyle choices or medical procedures. Priming yourself for conception has much more to do with what happens outside the bedroom than inside it. Look into your past to see if there is an incident that may have contributed to a tilted uterus. Remember, it doesn't have to be a situation in which you sustained serious injury. In fact, in most cases it isn't. Even if you can't recall one, it's essential to have your uterine alignment examined if you've had any trouble conceiving.

A qualified examination along with employing the best habits that support a fertile body and mind is the most effective way to eliminate fertility frustration. When we do this we are doubly blessed, not only with the birth of a healthy baby in most cases, but with the profound shift in consciousness that comes with experiencing one of the greatest gifts in life, giving life to another human soul.

Chapter 14

Perilous Prevention

Rethinking mammogram screening

Cancer is the second leading cause of death in the United States, so it's understandable that it gets a great deal of press coverage. The downside is that a lot of misperceptions about cancer get reinforced over time, and this generates fear. Because of this, the overall impression for most people seems to be that cancer is a death sentence and that it grows quickly. Generally speaking, both those assumptions are wrong.

Even so, the assumption that most cancers are fast-growing has led to the belief that early detection and fast treatment is the best defense. Unfortunately, this fear-driven approach to find even the smallest anomalies in tissue and treat them as mature diseases is leading patients to make treatment decisions they later regret. For women, nowhere is this phenomenon more prevalent than in the fight against breast cancer. At the same time, compelling evidence is showing that the early detection method we once saw as the gold standard for diagnosing breast cancer, the yearly mammogram, is less reliable than we once thought and worse, harming millions of women.

Misplaced Praise

Since the 1960s, the mammogram has been the most trusted method of breast cancer screening. If an irregularity was found, a woman could expect a biopsy and find herself in treatment within weeks or even days. After the ordeal, she could be grateful that her life was saved due to the fact that she acted quickly and that the mammogram caught the cancer in time. Mammograms were viewed then as they are now, nearly infallible. Radiologists, oncologists, and many cancer organizations will insist that mammograms have saved millions of lives because of early detection and intervention.

Today, research is showing that mammography's success rate is over-stated because, as a screening tool, it's much better at identifying slow-moving, non-aggressive cancers rather than the more serious kind. High survival statistics from millions of women who detected their cancer via mammogram aren't necessarily due to early detection but because their cancers were slow-growing and even dormant.

A Common Problem

A big reason for the inflated mammogram early detection survival rates is a common breast pathology known as ductal carcinoma in situ (DCIS). This condition, which affects a high percentage of women, often lays dormant in a woman's body her entire life. Incredibly, DCIS is now being called *stage zero* breast cancer. I can't even begin to explain that kind of reasoning.

DCIS has been the subject of many studies but the most interesting reviewed the autopsies of a wide cross-section of women. Researchers discovered that 40% of the women had DCIS present in their breast tissue at the time of death. These women had died from a wide range of causes, including car accidents. DCIS was even present in the breast tissue of women in advanced age. The point to understand here is that these women went on happily living their lives with no symptoms or awareness of their DCIS until they died of *something else.*[1][2]

Since 1980, DCIS has increased 300% and accounts for 25% of all early stage cancers detected by mammography.[3] The concern is that with DCIS being categorized as cancer and a four-fold increase in diagnosis in recent years, women are rushing into fear-based treatment decisions that they may regret later on. Sadly, that appears to be the case.

Epidemic of Overdiagnosis

A 2012 study published in *The New England Journal of Medicine* looked at breast cancer trends in women over 40 from 1976 to 2008. All breast pathologies were included from DCIS to late-stage cancers. The study made an interesting point. From the time mammography was introduced on a large scale in the United States, a *simultaneous doubling* of early-stage breast cancer diagnosis occurred. Before mammography was introduced, 122 women per 100,000 were diagnosed with early-stage breast cancers and after, 234. Once the researchers averaged out the women with late-stage cancers and those under 40, they came to this startling conclusion.

> …that breast cancer was over-diagnosed (i.e., tumors were detected on screening that would never have led to clinical symptoms) in 1.3 million U.S. women in the past 30 years. We estimated that in 2008 breast cancer was over-diagnosed in more than 70,000 women; this accounted for 31% of all breast cancers diagnosed.
>
> Despite substantial increases in the number of cases of early-stage breast cancer detected, screening mammography has only marginally reduced the rate at which women present with advanced cancer…and that screening is having, at best, only a small effect on the rate of death from breast cancer.[4]

This study got a lot of attention and has been instrumental in reducing the blind trust doctors and patients placed in mammograms for so long. There should never be a rush into serious treatment until all options have been discussed and especially when there is a strong likelihood that the condition will never advance to clinical symptoms. Sadly, millions of women in the past never got this advice and made drastic decisions for what were benign conditions.

A review team examined the records from a study performed at Yale-New Haven Hospital in 1988. The study followed 233 women who had their first experience with breast cancer. Examining the medical records, the reviewers found the prognosis for all the women was excellent. The reviewers came to this conclusion not because the cancers were detected early but because they were either slow-growing or dormant, requiring minimal treatment. Of the study participants, 31 were diagnosed with DCIS. The good news is that none died from cancer or experienced a recurrence. Unfortunately, half of them chose to have a mastectomy.[5]

Breaking with Tradition

In spite of these dramatic findings, national cancer organizations have been reluctant to let go of the early-detection-saves-lives assumption with regard to mammograms and breast cancer. The American Cancer Society (ACS) made slight changes to its previous recommendations. At present, it no longer recommends a yearly mammogram for women beginning at age 40 but 45. After 55, the recommendation is for a mammogram every two years.[6] It states this even though the ACS openly acknowledges in its mammogram guidelines the problem of over-diagnosing DCIS as cancer leading to over-treatment "because the cancer never would have caused any problems" and that this "exposes some women to the side effects of cancer treatment even though it wasn't really needed."[7]

Although the National Cancer Institute (NCI) does not issue cancer screening guidelines, it addresses the inconsistencies and risks associated with yearly mammograms. It states "Not all breast cancers will cause death or illness in a woman's lifetime, so they may not need to be found or treated." It admits that decisions about getting screenings can be "difficult" because "not all screening tests are helpful, and most have harms."[8]

Results & Radiation

One of those harms is ending up having an unnecessary painful biopsy because for every 10 women having a mammogram, one will get a false-positive. This naturally leads to the doctor ordering a biopsy. In fact, the more mammograms a woman has the higher her chances are of getting a false-positive. The NCI states that a woman getting a mammogram every year for 10 years increases her chance of getting a false-positive by more than 50% and yet, healthy women over 44 are still being told to get a yearly mammogram.[9]

Actually, most positive results turn out to *not* be cancer, especially for women who are under 50, had a previous biopsy, have a family history of breast cancer, or are taking hormones for menopause. Ultimately, the NCI recommends that whatever benefits mammography offers need to be "balanced against its harms" because over-diagnosis and having treatment for breast anomalies "that may never cause health problems or become life-threatening may cause serious side effects and may not lead to a longer, healthier life." They advise the decision to get a mammogram needs to be made between you and your doctor.[10] [11]

A Danish review of seven studies investigating mammograms agreed. Researchers found that mammograms didn't contribute to saving the lives of women in any way that could be supported by statistics. They also mentioned the volume of unwarranted medical interventions like biopsies that were routinely performed after mammograms and a 20% increase in mastectomies, most of which were unnecessary. It's no wonder the study was titled *Is screening for breast cancer with mammography justifiable?*[12]

Another concern with recurring mammograms for healthy women is the cumulative exposure to radiation which in itself is a risk factor for breast cancer, especially for women with large breasts or breast implants where higher doses of radiation are needed.[13] In fact, the average effective dose of radiation in one mammogram is four times greater than a chest x-ray.[14] Research has shown that biennial (every other year) mammograms do indeed raise the breast cancer risk in healthy women, and it's even higher for women with other risk factors.[15]

Cellular Detection

Fortunately, there's a nontoxic, pain-free, and more accurate way for women to have breast screenings. Thermography uses infrared imaging to measure heat activity inside the breast. All cancer starts with inflammation at the cellular level, and inflammation generates heat. It's also excellent at detecting increased blood flow to the breast because cancer needs additional nutrients to grow. New blood vessel growth also becomes visible, revealing new networks built specifically to support nourishment and growth for a developing tumor. The amazing aspect of thermography is that because it's looking for heat-related anomalies it can detect cancerous activity at the cellular level even before a viable tumor takes shape. In fact, thermography is so sensitive that studies have shown it can detect cancerous activity eight to 10 years before any other screening method.[16] In contrast, when a tumor is finally detectable through a mammogram or other type of screening, it's had a seven-year head start.

More than 800 peer-reviewed studies have been conducted on thermography, continually demonstrating its effectiveness, especially in detecting early cancerous activity which mammograms aren't as sensitive at recognizing. One study published by the *American Journal of Radiology* showed that thermography was 97% accurate in detecting breast cancers in women who'd previously had a suspicious mammogram. [17] Because of its accuracy rate, researchers have called thermography "an excellent primary method" of breast cancer screening in order to determine if a mammogram is necessary.[18] In fact, positive thermograms followed up by a necessary mammogram can detect 95% of early stage cancers.[19]

In other good news, thermography is pain-free because heat sensitive cameras simply scan the breasts and make no contact with them. Breast density, scar tissue, and implants do not hinder its accuracy because it isn't taking an x-ray of physical tissue which is also the reason it's completely non-toxic with zero radiation exposure. That means it's entirely safe for women who might be pregnant or breastfeeding.

What's Old Is New

Thermography sounds like a new invention, but it's been around since the 1940s. In 1982, it was FDA approved as an adjunct screening method for breast cancer. Why didn't you know about it? It's probably because the influence behind the radiology industry would prefer that you have mammograms. That's usually how these things go—follow the money. By equating DCIS with breast cancer and the consistent false positive rate, mammograms also generate a large revenue stream that supports surgeons and lab analysis as well as chemotherapy and radiation services.

When searching for an imaging center, you'll want to confirm that the drift factor of the equipment is no greater than 0.2 degrees Centigrade to provide the proper image clarity. Because this is a heat-sensitive procedure, the room shouldn't be warmer than about 72 degrees. The procedure should take place in a windowless room, and the scans should preferably be read on site, not sent out. The doctor should be the one to go over your results with you. Remember to confirm certifications and credentials. Most of the time, thermograms aren't covered by insurance. For more information on thermography, you can visit the Eagle Institute of Clinical Thermology at breastthermography.com and the International Academy of Clinical Thermology at iact-org.org.

I want to say that I'm not anti-mammogram only when they're unnecessary which tends to be much of the time. Why expose yourself to dangerous radiation, the inevitability and trauma of a false positive, and the painful biopsy that follows when there's a safer alternative? I would suggest using both thermogram and mammogram to your maximum advantage. Having a yearly thermogram is excellent and accurate healthcare prevention. If any irregularity presents itself on a thermogram, discuss with your doctor the possibility of following it up with a mammogram. That's breast cancer prevention performed properly.

Chapter 15

In One Basket

The false promise of frozen eggs for fertility

Brigitte Adams was on the top of the world. She was a graduate of Vassar College working in tech marketing for several prestigious international companies, spoke fluent Italian, and earned a multiple six-figure salary. In her 30s, her plan was to work a few more years then find Mr. Right and start a family. She contacted a fertility clinic, had a number of her eggs cryogenically frozen, and continued to climb the corporate ladder.

During this time, she became a national role model for modern female empowerment when she appeared on the cover of *Bloomberg Businessweek* in a power suit with briefcase in hand under the title Freeze your eggs, Free your career. The article celebrated Brigitte's success as proof that women could use modern technology to delay motherhood in favor of a career in their quest to "have it all."

Four years later, Mr. Right never arrived and Brigitte found herself scrambling to choose a sperm donor and thaw her frozen eggs in an attempt to have the baby she desperately wanted. Two eggs didn't survive the thawing process. Three failed to fertilize. Six embryos were declared abnormal. When the last embryo implanted into her uterus failed, Brigitte knew that being over 40 there was a near 0% chance of ever being able to have a child of her own. In an interview with the *Washington Post*, she described screaming "like a wild animal" throwing her books, papers, and laptop across the room, and collapsing to the floor.[1] By putting all her eggs and hopes in the promise of delaying motherhood with technology, she was bitterly disappointed.

Conquering the Fertility Clock?

For years, the media has trumpeted the praises of fertility technology, an industry aimed almost exclusively at women. Among all other procedures, the cryopreservation or freezing of eggs has received a disproportionate amount of attention or some might say promotion. Years ago, the headlines were everywhere implying that the female biological clock had finally been conquered: Motherhood on Your Own Terms, Take Control of Your Body Calendar, Extend Your Fertility, and Leave Conception for Later. The implication was that women could schedule motherhood as easily as they scheduled a client meeting or business trip. There was no need to worry about age anymore because eggs frozen at 30 would still be viable and healthy even in a 40-year-old body.

The truth is science is nowhere near conquering the fertility cycle of the female body and giving women the option to put off motherhood to middle age (35+) and beyond. So little has been achieved in fertility science that it can hardly be called a science at all. For example, it's been 49 years since the first baby was born through *in vitro* fertilization (IVF) and yet, there remains a 77% failure rate and that's for women under 35. If you're older, it's 91%.[2]

Healthy men remain fertile into their 80s because they produce millions of new sperm daily. In contrast, women are born with a finite number of eggs, all they will ever produce in their lifetime. The younger a woman is the more viable her eggs are and the odds are much greater that she will have a healthy baby through a relatively uncomplicated birth. Because of this and the fact that a woman's egg count starts to decrease with her first period around age 12, nature has designed women to have their children as early as possible with a relatively short fertility window peaking between the ages of 17 and 30. After 35, a woman's fertility rate drops significantly in what's known as the "fertility cliff", making conception more difficult and bringing with it new risks and possible complications because of abnormalities in her eggs and other issues. By 40, a woman has only a 5% chance of conceiving.[3]

These facts show it isn't possible for the vast majority of women to beat the fertility clock and delay motherhood into their late 30s and early 40s by freezing their eggs or through other means. While you might know a woman or celebrity who had a baby at 41, she is the rare exception rather than the rule. On the contrary, the fertility industry would like women to believe the exact opposite and that freezing their eggs is the way to beat Mother Nature and "extend" their fertility when there really is no way to do that. Unfortunately, this only makes billions of dollars for the fertility industry and leaves tens of thousands of women heartbroken and struggling with regret.

Harvesting Eggs...and Money

Normally, a woman's body releases one egg per month. In order to retrieve a larger number for freezing, a woman must first submit to an extensive series of blood tests, ultrasounds, and other examinations in the days or weeks leading up to the retrieval. During this time, she will be injecting herself with a powerful combination of hormones over a series of days in order to hyper-stimulate the ovaries to release larger numbers of eggs. It should be noted that some of the hormones used in this process are done so "off-label" meaning they have never been studied or intended for such use. Each harvest cycle of eggs costs around $20,000 with most women undergoing two cycles. Fertility clinics will charge approximately $1,000 per month storage fee.[4]

When the time comes to use her eggs, the woman must again inject herself with hormones in order to prepare the uterus to accept the embryo. Once again, a heavy protocol of blood tests, ultrasounds, vaginal probes, and other preparations lead up to the implantation. Up to 15% of eggs don't survive the thawing process. Because the sperm cannot penetrate the cold, hardened outer membrane of the egg, it must be injected directly inside through a process called intracytoplasmic sperm injection (ICSI). If any of the eggs fertilize successfully, they are monitored for five days with the most promising being transferred to the woman's womb through IVF which can cost about $12,000 even though the overwhelming majority of attempts fail ending in spontaneous miscarriage.

Failure & Fraud

A study published in the journal *Fertility and Sterility* confirmed the failure rate of 77% for embryo implantations using frozen eggs for women age 30.[5] According to the American Society for Reproductive Medicine (ASRM), the chances of just one frozen egg leading to a live birth in a woman under 38 is 2% to 12%.[6] As if those odds weren't sobering enough, the average age of American women freezing their eggs is 37.4.[7] Overall, fewer than 2,000 people were ever born from frozen eggs and only 10 of them have been born to women 38 or older. When asked about the effectiveness of frozen egg implantation, ASRM practice committee chair, Samantha Pfeifer stated, "That has not been evaluated in any randomized controlled studies."[8]

The fact that the effectiveness of using frozen eggs for conception has never been subjected to a legitimate research study should come as no surprise. Fertility clinics that make millions off of 30-something women do their best to keep the massive failure rates a closely guarded secret. Even so, when researchers contacted every fertility clinic in the U.S. about their success rates the responses, although limited, were very telling. In all, 64% of the clinics contacted responded. Of those 140 clinics, 45 had never even thawed their clients' eggs. Just over 30 achieved no live births from their thawed eggs while 11 achieved just one live birth. Only eight clinics said they achieved 10 or more live births.[9] In the UK, which tracks fertility outcomes through its Human Fertilisation and Embryology Authority (HFEA), only 20 people were ever born from frozen eggs.[10]

Even when the media reports the extremely low success rates for frozen eggs, it does so in a way that still leaves women with unrealistic expectations. The *Washington Post* article that told Brigitte Adams' story featured a graph from a 2017 study published in *Human Reproduction* that promoted the newest selling angle for freezing eggs: freeze more eggs at a younger age. The claim is that the younger the eggs are the greater the chances will be of success. The graph makes the claim that a woman under 35 who freezes 30 eggs will still have a 58% chance of conceiving by age 41. Of course, the fine print beneath the graph reads, "Study uses mathematical model based on extrapolated data, not real world percentages from live births."[11] A newer study making the same claim found women freezing more eggs earlier had a 38% success rate of live births if they were under 38 and a miraculous 29% success rate for women over 38, but the research was based heavily on a small study of just 167 women.[12]

The idea that eggs harvested earlier are more viable and stay "frozen" at the age they're retrieved is misleading. Time doesn't stop for frozen eggs. They continue to age too, albeit slower. Even so, no one seems to think that the woman's body continuing to age at a normal pace will create any obstacles to conception. All the focus is placed on the age of the egg. It's a typical reductionist approach of western medicine that looks only at isolated parts and never the whole. Putting a "young" egg into an older body is like trying to put new furniture into an old house and expecting everything to coordinate naturally. As a woman's body ages, her energy changes along with her. Physiologically, hormonally, and energetically she's not nearly as primed for pregnancy at 39 as she was at 22. Pregnancy is a whole-body function in women. It's not all about the egg, not by a long shot.

Dr. James A. Grifo, specialist at NYU Langone Health and one of the pioneers of egg freezing, called the idea of women being able to control their fertility promoted by the media and fertility industry "destructive."

"It's total fiction. It's incorrect," Grifo said. "Your whole life it's beaten into your head that you're in control…There has to be more dialogue about what women can be responsible for and what they are not responsible for."[13]

Risk Without Reward

In addition to the enormous failure rate, the entire process of retrieving and freezing eggs carries a number of known and unknown health risks for women and any rare embryo that happens to remain viable. Repeated injections of high amounts of hormones to increase egg release can lead to ovarian hyper-stimulation syndrome which causes nausea, bloating, and discomfort. Although rare, serious cases have occurred requiring hospitalization along with complications such as intra-abdominal bleeding, ovarian torsion, and severe pain.

According to the Center for Genetics and Society (CGS), there also remains concern about the long-term risks associated with using powerful hormone cocktails that contain hormones that were never medically approved for such purposes. Concerns have been raised about infertility, cancer, and the effects on any children born from frozen eggs because the chemicals used in the freezing process are known to be toxic. Unfortunately, long-term health studies on women using frozen eggs for conception have never been done. At the same time, women using frozen eggs must undergo IVF which has been linked to an increase in stillbirths, cesarean sections, preterm deliveries, multiple gestations, and higher rates of fetal anomalies.[14]

Reproductive endocrinologists have stated that physicians have a responsibility to accurately inform women of all the short and long-term risks associated with egg retrieval and implantation. Those risks include the "...potential for scar tissue formation around the ovaries and fallopian tubes...[that]...could interfere with future natural conception by preventing an otherwise normal egg from entering the fallopian tube after ovulation...For women looking to electively freeze their eggs, the process could worsen their chances of conceiving naturally."[15]

Aside from the physical risks, women using frozen eggs find themselves on an emotional rollercoaster. With every failure or miscarriage comes a tidal wave of feelings like sadness, anger, and especially regret that can be overwhelming. A study that interviewed 500 women ages 27 to 44 two years after using frozen eggs found that 50% experienced moderate to severe regret. Interestingly, the average age of the women was 36 with 80% holding a graduate degree and 70% earning over $100,000.[16] Researchers stated that using frozen eggs was "emotionally more complex than people might have assumed initially" and expressed shock that a significant percentage of the women "grossly overestimated" their probability of having a child with some believing the success rate was near 100%.[17]

Experts Refuse to Endorse

Much of the confusion and marketing around freezing eggs came after the ASRM removed the "experimental" label from the procedure. Almost immediately, fertility clinics began marketing the idea of controlling fertility and postponing motherhood to women. What they neglected to tell women was that the ASRM *only* approved of freezing eggs for younger women with cancer as a way to protect them from the effects of chemotherapy and to provide the patients with a very small opportunity of having a child later. Approving elective egg freezing for healthy women or even implying that it was effective for such use was never their intention.

ASRM committee chair Samantha Pfeifer stated, "While a careful review of the literature indicates egg freezing is a valid technique for young women for whom it is medically indicated, we cannot at this time endorse its widespread elective use to delay childbearing. This technology may not be appropriate for the older woman who desires to postpone reproduction."

She went on to say, "Marketing this technology for the purpose of deferring childbearing may give women false hope and encourage women to delay childbearing. Patients who wish to pursue this technology should be carefully counseled."[18]

The ASRM was joined by the Society for Assisted Reproductive Technology (SART) in publicly stating that freezing eggs should never be recommended to healthy women. The official statement said, "...there are not yet sufficient data to recommend oocyte cryopreservation for the sole purpose of circumventing reproductive aging in healthy women because there are no data to support the safety, efficacy, ethics, emotional risks, and cost-effectiveness of oocyte cryopreservation for this indication."[19] After the article was published, the American College of Obstetricians and Gynecologists (ACOG) publicly declared they also would not endorse egg freezing for healthy women as an effective way to delay motherhood.[20]

Corporate Conniving

The fact that the ASRM, SART, and ACOG all came out publicly against egg freezing as ineffective and possibly unsafe for healthy women didn't stop companies like Meta (Facebook) and Apple from adding it to health benefits packages. The companies offered $20,000 to all female employees who chose to freeze their eggs. The decision released a firestorm of criticism. The accusation was that the companies only offered such a benefit in order to convince women to delay motherhood, keeping them on the job years longer so the company could avoid having to deal with the issues that come with pregnant employees. In the end, it was a policy that worked to benefit the companies and not the women who would only end up disappointed years later when their frozen eggs almost certainly failed.

An official statement from CGS, a nonprofit agency that advocates for responsible use and oversight of reproductive and genetics biotechnology, criticized the alleged benefit to women. In a scathing indictment it stated that instead of encouraging women to delay motherhood so they could work longer, the Silicon Valley companies should have been focused on creating new policies for paid leave and schedule flexibility that would enable work-family balance for women.

CGS executive director Marcy Darnovsky added, "Paying for egg freezing is being presented as a benefit for women, but it may be that discouraging women from balancing work and family is really a benefit to the companies."[21] She later added, "When you're in a situation of your employer offering you a choice, you really have to be careful that you're distinguishing between something that's an expanded option and something that's actually subtle or even explicit pressure to do what your employer wants you to do."[22]

Online, the outcry from women was just as loud. One woman spoke for many when she called corporate egg freezing incentives "a sign your workplace is a dystopian hellhole" bluntly stating, "This is the kind of woman empowerment that makes me cringe. But if there is anything I've learned working in tech for almost a decade, it's that this is par for the course. That corporate feminism like 'Lean In' (by Facebook's COO) isn't about making women's lives better; it's about increasing our productivity for the good of the company."[23]

The best chance any woman has at conceiving and having healthy babies is to have them as early as possible. Of course, that timeline can vary greatly from one woman to another. Money can be an obstacle to starting a family as is the time it takes to find a good mate. Even so, young people must find creative ways to overcome these challenges if they wish to have families because nature doesn't change and time moves on.

We must help young people rearrange their priorities and once again place more importance on family and relationships. Motherhood is the most important and rewarding job a woman will ever have. That doesn't mean young women shouldn't pursue careers. It simply means that work will always be there but their fertility won't, and it's very dangerous to put all their eggs and hope for motherhood in one basket.

Chapter 16

A Blind Eye

How the HPV vaccine harms female fertility

Vaccine safety and efficacy have been hot button issues since the 1980s when the recommended vaccine schedule for children began to climb dramatically, up from five shots of three vaccines in 1962 to 24 shots of five vaccines in 1983. Today it's 72 shots of 13 vaccines. As children began receiving more vaccines, the autism rate increased right along with it and concerned parents and health officials started asking questions. Soon after in 1986, Congress passed the Childhood Vaccination Injury Act that gave pharmaceutical companies producing vaccines full federal protection from lawsuits. It led many people to ask if vaccines were really safe why their makers needed protection from liability.

Although the CDC was ordered by Congress in 1986 to determine if vaccines like DTP, DTaP, Hep B, HIB, PCV 13 and IPV caused autism, the National Academy of Medicine which was charged with supervising the CDC in this regard confirmed years later[1] that the research was never done.[2] The only vaccine ever studied with regard to autism was the MMR vaccine, and during a reanalysis of the data researchers found a statistically significant connection between the vaccine and autism, particularly among African American male infants.[3] The research created a firestorm of criticism from the medical industry and media and was later retracted by the journal that published it. Even so, other scientists from the Department of Health and Human Services (HHS) have submitted sworn affidavits to the Department of Justice confirming the vaccines/autism connection.[4]

Even now, as the autism rate in America has exploded from less than three in 10,000[5] to one in 36 today[6] the CDC still maintains that vaccines are safe and do not cause autism.[7] Strangely, the CDC makes this claim while spending tens of millions of dollars tracking a few hundred cases of measles, an illness that kills virtually no one, while turning a blind eye to the epidemic of 68,000 new cases of autism diagnosed each year without conducting any large scale, long-term studies on vaccines and autism.[8]

At the same time, researchers in the World Health Organization's (WHO) African vaccine program found that children receiving the DTP vaccine had a mortality rate 10 times higher than children who were unvaccinated. It was found that the vaccine had weakened the children's immune system so severely that they died in droves from unrelated infections. The researchers concluded, "The DTP vaccine may kill more children from other causes than it saves from diphtheria, tetanus and pertussis."[9]

Unhealthy Investment

The greatest concern with asking government agencies to research vaccine safety is that many of them, including those created to improve and protect our health, have significant conflicts of interest when it comes to such research. The Food and Drug Administration (FDA) receives 45% of its annual budget from the pharmaceutical industry. The WHO gets 50% of its budget from private sources, including the pharmaceutical industry and its allied foundations. The CDC holds the patents for 56 vaccines while buying and distributing $4.6 billion in vaccines each year through its Vaccines for Children Program which represents 40% of its budget.[10] HHS partners with vaccine makers to develop, approve, recommend, and pass mandates for new vaccines. In fact, HHS employees receive up to $150,000 per year in royalties from vaccines they work on.[11] This enormous financial incentive for government healthcare agencies is precisely why, after vaccine makers were freed from all liability in 1986, the vaccine schedule for children now includes 11 times more shots than a few decades ago, exemptions are being eliminated, and vaccination has exploded into a $50 billion industry.[12]

Absence of Standards

Free from liability and with a market of 76 million U.S. children mandated to be vaccinated for school, there is zero incentive for vaccine makers to ensure their products are safe. Only four companies, Merck, GSK, Sanofi, and Pfizer make most vaccines and they've collectively paid over $35 billion in fines for defrauding regulators, bribing government officials and physicians, and falsifying scientific data about products that they told us were safe and effective.[13] It is any wonder people are skeptical when they're told vaccines are safe?

Because vaccines are so lucrative for manufacturers and government health agencies, they are often "fast-tracked" through the FDA rigorous safety testing before being licensed and released for public use. While other drugs are typically required to go through five to 10 years of double-blind, controlled studies, vaccines are often approved in a much shorter time period. For the COVID-19 vaccines, it was only 11 months.[14] [15]

Even worse, vaccines are not tested against an inert placebo such as a shot of saline solution. When two drugs are tested against each other, especially if they have similar ingredients and no placebo is in place, it's impossible to discover which components might be causing adverse effects because nothing has been isolated. There is no capacity to assess a medication's risk. It's also impossible to determine a medication's effectiveness because in order to be deemed effective by FDA standards a medication must perform better than a placebo.

Safety for Sale

Adding to the lack of safety protocol, a report from the National Academy of Medicine (NAM) found that there has *never* been a single study comparing the differences in health outcomes between vaccinated and unvaccinated children. Equally, studies examining the long-term health effects of cumulative vaccines or other aspects of the vaccine schedule "have not been conducted."[16] Approving vaccines within a matter of weeks or months doesn't allow enough time to identify and track many illnesses that vaccinated children often present with later on such as allergies, asthma, autoimmune diseases, cancer, seizure disorders, arthritis, diabetes, rhinitis, neurological disorders, autism, and hundreds of other injuries listed on manufacturers' inserts. It seems more than coincidental that before the vaccine schedule exploded in 1986 12.8% of American children suffered from chronic diseases.[17] Today, it's 54%.[18]

If vaccines worked the way they are claimed, the U.S. should have the healthiest children because we have the most aggressive vaccine schedule in the world. Unfortunately, since the mid-1980s, health outcomes for American children have plummeted, ranking 35th behind Costa Rica,[19] giving us the sickest children and the highest infant mortality in the developed world.[20]

Because virtually no safety research has been done on vaccines, vaccination advocates almost always have to rely on appeals to authority such as the CDC, FDA, or WHO that state vaccines are safe in order to support their claims instead of scientific evidence. Even more, NAM, which was designated by HHS as monitor of the CDC's vaccine safety research, has stated that the claims of these agencies are entirely unfounded because the necessary research simply hasn't been done and which the CDC still refuses to perform.[21]

In spite of this, NAM has released several investigative reports[22] determining that more than 30 conditions have a causal connection to vaccines.[23] In examining the tiny amount of data the CDC has produced over decades, NAM stated that is was so inadequate it couldn't possibly be used to accept or reject vaccine causation.

In the meantime, the National Vaccine Injury Compensation Program at HHS has paid out more than $5 billion in compensation to Americans injured by vaccines.[24] This seems to be a telling admission because if vaccines were proven to be safe, they wouldn't be paying anyone.

Although the CDC refuses to do vaccine safety research, it has set up the Vaccine Adverse Event Reporting System (VAERS), an online information portal where vaccine injuries can be self-reported and tabulated by vaccine, type of injury, and year. In 2023, the system received 105,333 reports of adverse events that included 864 deaths, 511 permanent disabilities, and 6,411 hospitalizations. In 2021, the system received its highest counts ever with 748,810 adverse events, 9,226 deaths, 11,005 permanent disabilities, and 44,194 hospitalizations.[25] Unfortunately, these numbers are just a tiny portion of the real impact because HHS has stated that less than 1% of vaccine injuries are ever reported.[26] This is largely due to the CDC's refusal to either mandate or automate reporting for healthcare providers, so it's left up to patients—if they are even aware of vaccine dangers—to self-report.

The media is reluctant to report these facts because it receives over $5 billion in advertising from the pharmaceutical industry each year.[27] All the while, the pharmaceutical companies make billions more from children who must take numerous medications like Adderall, asthma inhalers, and ADHD and anti-seizure medicines because of vaccine-related illnesses for the rest of their lives.

Selling Fear

The most recent vaccine-related childhood health tragedy comes to us by way of the HPV vaccine which is said to protect against the human papilloma virus that has been linked to cervical cancer. HPV is the most common sexually transmitted disease and presently affects 79 million Americans.[28] There are about 100 different strains with all but a few being harmless. The most common is associated with genital warts, which aren't dangerous, and can be removed with a minor procedure. The virus is transferred through skin-to-skin contact, usually via the mouth, genitals, and other sexual areas of the body. This makes it very easy to contract which is why so many people have already been exposed.

Sold as Gardasil by Merck in the U.S. and as Cervarix by GSK in Europe, the CDC approved the HPV vaccine three-shot series for girls between 11 and 26. With a fear-based ad campaign, pharmaceutical companies and the CDC urged parents to vaccinate their children against HPV before they became sexually active to protect against the miniscule risk of dying from cervical cancer. Strangely, the vaccine is also approved for boys.

According to the CDC, six million women contract HPV each year, but only 4,000 of them will die from cervical cancer, mostly due to not getting regular pap smears.[29] To put this in perspective, just 0.0007% of women contracting HPV annually will die from cervical cancer and even less if they see their gynecologist regularly.

The CDC claims that 37,000 Americans are diagnosed with HPV related cancers each year. In reaching this number, the CDC explained that its researchers simply added up the numbers of cases where cancer occurred in parts of the body where HPV is commonly found, *not* whether those cancers were actually caused by HPV. In fact, the CDC admits that the cancer registries researchers used to make this claim "do not routinely collect data on whether HPV is in the cancer tissue."[30] Then it's impossible to know if HPV played a role in any of those cancers.

Truth & Tragedy

The truth is HPV is virtually harmless with only two strains (16 and 18) out of 100 considered to be high risk. Even in those cases, research has consistently shown[31] that the body will naturally eradicate HPV[32] on its own in 90% of cases.[33] The odds are even better if the person is under age 30. When interviewed by *SELF* magazine about HPV, board certified gynecologists stated, "The vast majority of people with HPV get rid of the virus naturally…Most [HPV infections] are self-limiting and will be self-cleared."[34]

Even the CDC admits on its own website, "More than 90% of new HPV infections, including those caused by high-risk HPV types, clear or become undetectable within two years, and clearance usually occurs in the first six months after infection."[35] It's an astonishing admission, so why the hysteria?

Condoms can prevent 70% of HPV infections.[36] Coupled with a greater than 90% chance of clearing by the immune system and regular pap smears, who needs a vaccine for what's essentially a non-lethal virus?

In spite of this information, the HPV vaccine is still aggressively promoted, especially to young girls. As with other vaccines, it's also implicated in an increasing number of adverse events, disabling injuries, and deaths.

At the time of this writing, a search of the VAERS database for all versions of the HPV vaccine returned 58,217 adverse events reported between the vaccine's release in 2006 through 2023. This included 2,066 hospitalizations, 1,529 permanent disabilities, and 259 deaths. This doesn't include other categories such as emergency room visits, life-threatening events, extended hospital stays, or birth defects/anomalies.[37]

Reproductive Ramifications

Of equally great concern is a growing number of young women who are experiencing premature ovarian failure (POF) approximately three years after receiving the HPV vaccine. POF is an extremely rare condition where the eggs in the ovaries spontaneously die and a woman immediately goes into menopause. At that point, she is infertile regardless of her age. Medical journals have been documenting[38] this rare phenomenon happening more often to girls as young as 16 who received the HPV vaccine around age 12.[39] Most reported seeing their menstrual cycle become increasingly irregular starting at six months after vaccination until menstruation completely stopped about two years later. As this shocking occurrence becomes more common in young women, medical investigators have urged rigorous inquiry into the subject.

The threat of POF after HPV vaccination received broader public awareness when sisters Madelyne and Olivia Meylor of Wisconsin both experienced POF at 16 and 17. After diagnostic testing, including genetic testing, couldn't provide answers, they filed a lawsuit against HHS.[40] A federal judge later threw the case out on a technicality and without making any determination as to the relationship between POF and the HPV vaccine.[41]

Around the same time the Meylor sisters filed their lawsuit, more than 2,000 Japanese women were reporting severe adverse reactions six months to three years after getting the HPV vaccine, including long-term pain, numbness, paralysis, and sudden unexplained infertility. As reports continued to grow, the Japanese Health Labor and Welfare Ministry withdrew support for the HPV vaccine and no longer recommends it.[42]

Preventing Pregnancies

For women who received the HPV vaccine but did not experience POF, studies are showing they have difficulty conceiving and become pregnant less often than unvaccinated women. A study of eight million women ages 25 to 29 found that 60% of the women who did not receive the HPV vaccine were pregnant at least once during the seven year study period, while only 35% of women that got the vaccine had conceived. Among married women, 75% who did not receive the HPV vaccine had conceived. In comparison, 50% of married women who'd received the shot had been pregnant. Because the HPV vaccine is a three-shot series, it was found that having just one of the shots without the others made a woman less likely to conceive than a woman who'd received none. The lead researcher, Gayle DeLong, stated:

> Results suggest that females who received the HPV shot were less likely to have ever been pregnant than women in the same age group who did not receive the shot. If 100% of females in this study had received the HPV vaccine, data suggest the number of women having ever conceived would have fallen by 2 million. Further study into the influence of HPV vaccine on fertility is thus warranted.[43]

The study went on to show that not only are birth rates for American women under 30 at record lows dropping 11.5% but that the sharp downturn began just one year after the HPV vaccine was licensed for public use in 2006. This was after a steady increase in births of 8.5%. Also noted were examinations of other studies documenting 48 cases of ovarian damage, 214 spontaneous abortions, 130 occurrences of amenorrhea (cessation of menstruation), and 123 cases of irregular menstruation.

The study went to great lengths to try and explain the drastic reduction in births for women under 30 by means other than the HPV vaccine. Abortions actually declined during the study period. Use of contraception remained static for that timeframe, and the effectiveness of contraceptive devices was unchanged. While the economic recession of 2008 was followed by a decrease in births, the economy was recovering by 2010. U.S. employment rates and birth rates tend to move together, however, as employment rates began to recover in 2010 births continued to decline. The study concluded:

> Data suggest that at least part of the reason for the recent decline in U.S. birth rates amongst females aged 25–29 may be associated with increasing injection of the HPV vaccine.

Scientific Sabotage

The study also called into question the methodology of the original Gardasil safety testing for a reason as to why the connection between the HPV vaccine and infertility problems was never made. In one of the tests, over 50% of the girls were too young (9 to 12) to examine abnormal changes in the menstrual cycle. In another, older girls were required to use birth control pills, making it impossible to track effects on fertility. Follow-ups only included adverse effects that happened in the two weeks following vaccination when research consistently shows major adverse events happen within 2 to 3 years after receiving the shots.

Even worse, the control group in some of the clinical trials received solutions containing some of the same substances already in the vaccine instead of plain saline solution. In other research, these substances were found to have side effects, including ovarian damage. Corrupting the placebo this way would falsely make the HPV vaccine appear no more risky than the placebo and at least as safe and effective. Clearly, the safety trials for the HPV vaccine constitute scientific misconduct if not fraud.

The study that presented these findings received a fierce backlash from the medical and pharmaceutical industries. Like the study connecting autism and vaccines, it was retracted several weeks later by the editor of the journal that published it.[44] The researcher responded with her own rebuttal defending her study shortly after.[45]

In the wake of the evidence of potential damage to fertility from the HPV vaccine, the American College of Pediatricians (ACP) issued a press release in 2016 publicly admitting it had concerns about the connection. It acknowledged:

- Long term ovarian function was not assessed in either the original rat safety studies or in the human vaccine trial.

- Potential mechanisms of action have been postulated based on autoimmune associations with the aluminum adjuvant used and previously documented ovarian toxicity in rats from another component, polysorbate 80.

- Since licensure of Gardasil in 2006, there have been about 213 VAERS reports involving amenorrhea, POF or premature menopause, 88% of which have been associated with Gardasil.

The ACP also announced that it was establishing a Vaccine Safety Datalink POF study to address these connections. It added that it would likely be years before results could be determined.[46]

Birth Control Vaccines

With so many young women suffering unusual fertility problems after vaccination, most people don't know that the WHO does indeed have a Task Force on Birth Control Vaccines. They have been working on contraceptive vaccines for decades and have spoken openly about their use across the world and in research since the early 1990s.

> Our study provides insights into possible modes of action of the birth control vaccine promoted by the Task Force on Birth Control Vaccines of the WHO (World Health Organization).
> ...we initiated studies relating to possible mechanisms of action and potential side effects of this vaccine, which should be relevant to world-wide regulation of population growth.[47]

One of the mechanisms being used in vaccines to reduce human births is the inclusion of human chorionic gonadotropin (hCG) coupled with a toxin such as HPV, tetanus, diphtheria, etc. to trigger an autoimmune response to the body's increased production of the hormone. After a female egg is fertilized by sperm and an embryo starts to develop, a woman's body begins to produce more hCG. This is the signal that tells the female body it is pregnant and triggers the rest of the hormonal cascade and biological changes. The body of a woman who had received a birth control vaccine would not only contain antibodies to the toxin but also antibodies to hCG that was coupled with it. Because of this, hCG would be seen as an invader and neutralized by the immune system as soon as the embryo begins to develop. Without the signal of hCG to tell the woman's body it's pregnant, the embryo will be swept out with her next menstrual cycle. Researchers have stated:

> Three major approaches to contraceptive vaccine development are being pursued at the present time. The most advanced approach...involves the induction of immunity against human chorionic gonadotrophin (hCG). Vaccines are being engineered ... incorporating tetanus or diphtheria toxoid linked to a variety of hCG-based peptides ... Clinical trials have revealed that such preparations are capable of stimulating the production of anti-hCG antibodies...
>
> The fundamental principle behind this approach to contraceptive vaccine development is to prevent the maternal recognition of pregnancy by inducing a state of immunity against hCG, the hormone that signals the presence of the embryo to the maternal endocrine system.
>
> In principle, the induction of immunity against hCG should lead to a sequence of normal, or slightly extended, menstrual cycles during which any pregnancies would be terminated... [Additional vaccines] aim to prevent conception by interfering with the intricate cascade of interactive events that characterize the union of male and female gametes at fertilization.[48]

There are over 50 journal articles on contraceptive[49] and anti-fertility vaccines.[50] It's research like this that has caused healthcare professionals in countries such as Kenya, [51] the Philippines, Nicaragua, and Brazil to become suspicious of large-scale vaccination campaigns conducted there by global organizations.[52]

It has never been stated that the HPV vaccine contains hCG. Even so, it does contain Polysorbate-80, a surfactant that reduces the surface tension between the boundaries of two liquids, a gas and a liquid, or a solid and a liquid. Pharmacology uses surfactants to deliver certain drugs through the blood-brain barrier, whose job is to protect the brain by keeping most things out. Research has found that exposure to Polysorbate-80 decreases the weight of the uterus and ovaries and causes chronic estrogenic stimulation. Studies with mice have shown affected ovaries are also impaired with regard to secreting progesterone and have degenerative follicles.[53]

The manufacturer's insert of other vaccines, including the flu vaccine, states that the shot "...has not been evaluated for carcinogenic or mutagenic potential or impairment of fertility." In the case of pregnant women receiving a vaccine, the insert states there is limited to no data available on the risk to an existing pregnancy, the safety of breastfeeding, or the quality of breast milk.[54]

Reversing Positive Health Trends

Although the HPV vaccine is purported to protect against cervical cancer, statistics show cervical cancer rates were in sharp decline in all countries where pap smear screening was used regularly for a total global decrease of 30% between 1989 and 2007 before the vaccine was in use. Some of the most dramatic declines per 100,000 were seen in Australia (13.5 to 7), France (11 to 7.1) and the U.S. (10.7 to 6.6).[55] Several years after the HPV vaccine was introduced in 2006 this trend was reversed, particularly in countries where vaccine campaigns were aggressive and a large percentage of young girls were vaccinated.

In the UK where 85% of girls between 14 and 18 were vaccinated, national statistics showed an increase of 70% in the rate of cervical cancer for these women when they reached 20 to 25 from 2.7 to 4.6 per 100,000. Women 25 to 30 who received the vaccine when they were 18 to 23 saw their cervical cancer rate increase 100% from 11 to 22. Women 25 to 34 who were exposed to less of the vaccine with only the catch-up shot saw their risk increase by 18% from 17 to 20.

Unvaccinated women in all age groups continued to see their cervical cancer rates decrease. This has been the case in all countries where vaccination rates were over 80% including Sweden, Australia, Norway, and others.[56] Even though 4.6 in 100,000 is still fairly low for women 20 to 25 in the UK, risk increases of 70% to 100% just 10 years after the HPV vaccine was introduced and in such a young age group after decades of decline is a phenomenon that should not be ignored.

In the U.S. where the HPV vaccine isn't mandatory, coverage rates of young women average about 60%. Because of this, the cervical cancer rate among all women under 50 has remained relatively stable from 7.4 in 2007 to 6.9 in 2021. The odds are great that if only vaccinated women were isolated from this group, we would see increases in cervical cancer rates similar to those seen in Europe.[57]

Cervical Cancer Concerns

In Sweden, where 80% of 12-year-old girls received the HPV vaccine and 60% between 13 and 18, cervical cancer cases increased 50% between 2006 and 2015, from 202 per 100,000 to 317. These shocking statistics prompted a Swedish researcher to publish a study examining how the HPV vaccine may actually cause cervical cancer and not protect against it in many women. The study also stated the researchers of the original HPV trials were aware of this risk but chose not to disclose it.

Out of 100 HPV strains, the HPV vaccine is said to protect against just four of them two of which, 16 and 18, have been associated with most cervical cancer. In a review of the original vaccine trials, the 2018 Swedish study found that the vaccine is only effective against strains 16 and 18 in women who have not been previously exposed. In women already carrying those strains, no new antibodies are produced by vaccination and therefore, no protection is provided.

The study found that in women who were previously exposed to HPV 16 or 18 and later received the vaccine, the 16 and 18 viral strains in the serum reactivated and accelerated the virus in their bodies, causing cell proliferation and higher rates of cancer. In addition, data showed it can cause reactivation of other "non-target" viruses in the body, including other HPV strains.[58]

Of equal concern is that young girls are not screened for which HPV strains they may have already been exposed to before vaccination. Since it is passed through skin-to-skin contact, being sexually active isn't a prerequisite for exposure. Children can be exposed by passing through their mother's birth canal. It seems anyone even contemplating the HPV vaccine should be pre-screened and if they discover they're carrying strain 16 or 18 should definitely consult with their doctor before receiving the shot. A regular pap smear can provide this simple information. Even so, we must remember in over 90% of women, the body will neutralize all HPV strains anyway, including 16 and 18.

Revelations & Retraction

As with the studies mentioned earlier linking vaccines to autism and the HPV vaccine with infertility, the Swedish study linking the HPV vaccine with cervical cancer was eventually retracted by the journal that published it. Anticipating a backlash to his findings, the researcher chose to publish his study under a pseudonym, explaining to the journal editors his need to avoid consequences to his career. Even though the editors were aware of the researcher's real identity, they retracted the article because of the alleged "deception" involved, not because the data was incorrect.[59]

In spite of the retraction of the Swedish study, a connection between cervical cancer and the HPV vaccine continues to be made. Among 305,000 adverse events that included 445 deaths, a study in the *British Medical Journal* attributed over 1,000 cancerous tumors, including 168 cervical cancers, to the HPV vaccine. Researchers stated:

> A healthy 16-year-old is at zero immediate risk of dying from cervical cancer but is faced with a small but real risk of death or serious disability from a vaccine that has yet to prevent a single case of cervical cancer.[60]

While the HPV vaccine isn't believed to contain hCG, it has been found in other vaccines where components of it have been shown to stimulate and increase the growth of resistant cancers, including cervical cancer.[61] This is of particular concern because researchers working on anti-fertility vaccines have previously stated interest in developing vaccines with regard to hCG sensitive cancers. Researchers stated:

> At the present time, studies are focused on increasing the immunogenicity and efficacy of the birth control vaccine, and examining its clinical applications in various hCG-producing cancers.[62]

Education & Understanding

With an adverse event rate of one in 15 including reproductive damage, autoimmune disease, cancer, and a death rate of 14 in 10,000, the HPV vaccine, like other vaccines, remains controversial.[63] The overall risk of dying of cervical cancer in the U.S. is 2.3 in 100,000, but the chances of getting an autoimmune disease from the HPV vaccine are 2.3 in 100. That's a risk 1,000 times greater than dying of cervical cancer.[64]

Always consult your doctor before getting any vaccine, especially if you are a young woman with plans to start a family or who is currently pregnant or breastfeeding. Get regular pap tests every three years with an HPV screening every five years. Most of all, understanding the body's innate ability to heal itself will go a long way toward making these important healthcare decisions.

Chapter 17

Balancing Act

The ups and downs of hormone therapy for women

For men, unless a chronic disease process or an exposure to toxins is involved, hormones remain at healthy levels and gradually decline over a lifetime. On the other hand, women must face menopause, a more immediate and distinct decline in hormone levels over as little as five to 10 years. Needless to say, this kind of rapid hormonal decline often creates symptoms that run the gamut from irritable to debilitating. It's during this difficult time that some women may need hormone therapy (HT) to regain their peace of mind and quality of life.

The point of HT should always be to remove symptoms, not elevate hormone levels to those of a 25-year-old. The hormonal cascade requires a very delicate balance, and the introduction of exogenous hormones, those obtained from outside the body, can wreak havoc on health without the proper knowledge and precision of application.

Understanding Menopause

At any given time, there are about 50 million women in the U.S. between the ages of 42 and 58 going through the change of life we call menopause.[1] The biggest misconception about menopause is that women are in it for years. Actually, menopause is only the woman's last menstrual cycle or period. In Greek, it means *meno* (month) and *pausis* (to cease). The average age of menopause for women is 51 after which time their ovulation cycle stops and they are considered postmenopausal.

It's mainly the five to 10 years leading up to menopause that gets the most attention and causes all the trouble. It's known as the perimenopausal period or perimenopause. Here is where women experience widely varying degrees of a host of symptoms that include hot flashes, insomnia, mood swings, memory loss, depression, night sweats, loss of libido, joint pain, dry skin, fatigue, rapid heartbeat, frequent urination, concentration problems, and weight gain. The severity of these symptoms often depends on a woman's biological constitution and the type of introduction she has had into perimenopause.

If she's in good health with no disease processes, a woman's symptoms should begin in her 40's and progress naturally which may or may not require HT. Women with chronic or autoimmune disease and sometimes those who over-exercise are usually forced into perimenopause early in their mid-30's resulting in a more intense experience that often requires HT. About 1% of women reach menopause before age 40.[2] Abrupt entries into menopause either through chemotherapy, radiation, or hysterectomy always cause severe symptoms that require HT.

Boom & Bust

As we know it today, HT didn't come into existence until the late 1960s. When Dr. Robert Wilson's book *Feminine Forever* was released in 1968, it became an instant sensation. In it, he described how estrogen treatment could benefit women's health and wellbeing through midlife. By the early 1970s, 28 million women would be taking the estrogen drug Premarin. The name was created from the origin of the estrogen, pregnant (pre) mare (mar) urine (in). Yes, that's pregnant horse's urine. The HT revolution was short-lived when in 1975 the *New England Journal of Medicine* published research that stated women taking estrogen increased their risk for uterine cancer by 400%.[3] After this made headlines, half of the women who were taking Premarin quit immediately.

In the 1980s, it became clear it was crucial that any women taking estrogen who still had a uterus needed to take progesterone as well to prevent hyperplasia, the thickening of the uterine lining that can lead to cancer. About the same time, the first synthetic progesterone drug, Provera, was released as an estrogen/synthetic progesterone (progestin) combo called Prempro.

Clearing the Air

Over the years, there has been much confusion concerning HT and its relation to increasing cardiovascular disease and cancer risk in women. Fortunately, there has been just as much research in the more than 50 years since HT began and the air is finally beginning to clear. In short, HT can protect women from cardiovascular disease, and the only measurable risk for breast cancer lies with conventional HT, which is negligible at that.

Research has shown that women who start estrogen-only HT within a decade after menopause experience an 11% to 30% reduction in heart attack risk. The earlier HT is begun the larger the benefit with the youngest women receiving a 44% risk reduction.[4] A periodic review of the famous Nurse's Health Study has shown similar results.[5]

The real cardiovascular risk comes with women over age 60 who already have a history of cardiovascular disease and begin taking Prempro (estrogen and progestin) for the first time. These women show a legitimate increase in heart attacks, artery blockages, and even gall bladder disease. It is not recommended that these women utilize HT. If, however, a healthy woman begins HT earlier in life she can expect no problems as she passes into her 60s and beyond.[6]

With regard to breast cancer risk, a follow-up review of the Women's Health Initiative (WHI) study found that women taking Prempro had a higher rate of invasive breast cancer and mortality than the placebo group, but this amounted to an increase of only 1.3 women in every 10,000.[7] To demonstrate how small this risk increase is the percentage comparison would be 0.34% for the placebo group and 0.42% for the HT group, just eight one-hundredths of a percent. It should also be noted that although the media likes to keep American women's attention focused on breast cancer, it's not the number one cancer killer for women. That's lung cancer.[8]

Conventional Hormone Options

Because Premarin, the most common form of conventional estrogen, is made from the urine of pregnant horses it can be problematic when introduced into the human body. Breaking it down, Premarin is estrone sulfate (>50%), equilin (15% to 25%) and equilenin. These *conjugated* estrogens are called as such because they are not in the true molecular form as a woman's own estrogen. Because of this, there is some concern over the equine (horse) estrogens in Premarin, particularly equilin and equilenin and how the body metabolizes them. Research published in *The Proceedings of the Society for Experimental Biology and Medicine*[9]and *Chemical Research and Toxicology*[10]showed that the body breaks these equine hormones down into metabolites that have an even stronger estrogenic effect than the horse estrogens themselves. They can create DNA damage in tissue that has been shown to be carcinogenic.[11] This is likely the reason why studies show a very small increase in cancer risk in women on conventional HT. It should also be noted that because most prescription drugs like Premarin need to be heavily metabolized by the body, they raise insulin levels.

Real progesterone doesn't have a long half-life. Because of that, the pharmaceutical companies needed something that lasted much longer so they created medroxyprogesterone acetate (MPA) also known as progestin. It was created at the same time as the birth control pill because in low regular doses it prevents ovulation.

While estrogen has been shown to protect women against heart disease, synthetic progesterone or progestin (Provera) can cancel out that benefit. When the WHI data was reviewed, women on Prempro (combination Premarin and Provera) did show an increase in myocardial infarctions and deaths from coronary artery disease and blood clots in the first two years on HT.[12]

A woman's body also produces testosterone. Although it's only a tiny amount, testosterone is also essential for women's health and libido and while rare may need to be included in HT treatment. Methyltestosterone is a completely synthetic form of testosterone and has been around for over 50 years. As an anabolic steroid, it's the most common type used by bodybuilders. It has a low bioavailability and is widely known for its negative cardiovascular effects and damaging the liver.[13] Aside from these more serious issues, all conjugated and synthetic (conventional) hormones come with a host of side effects because they are not truly natural and will elicit a defensive response of some kind from the body.

Bioidentical Hormone Options

Bioidentical hormones are called as such because they are *identical* in molecular structure to the estrogen, progesterone, and testosterone found in the human body. They are the exact same hormones the body uses, making their bioavailability very high and side effects virtually non-existent. Identical means they are an *exact match*, unlike the label of "natural" which can be used to include many substances that might be from nature but are foreign to the human body.

Plants have hormonal properties just like humans and in the 1930s it was discovered that a plant steroid, diosgenin, found in yams could easily be converted into an exact match for human progesterone using only heat and pressure, no chemicals. Bioidentical testosterone also comes from yams.

In the same way, bioidentical estrogen is derived from soybeans. If you're concerned about the negative effects of soy as part of the diet, there's no need to panic here. After the conversion process, none of the phyto (plant-based) estrogen properties remain in place. It's not similar to human estrogen; it's *identical.* The plant-based estrogen structure no longer exists.

Myth Busting

Bioidentical hormones are the exact substances that the body creates so unlike conventional hormones, they cannot be patented. Because of this, pharmaceutical corporations can't make any money off of them. That's why all the large longitudinal studies have always focused on synthetic and conventional hormones like Premarin and Prempro. It's also the reason why drug companies are often not honest when talking about bioidentical hormones.

The biggest misconception they perpetuate is that bioidentical hormones are not FDA regulated. Regulation simply means that the

FDA guarantees their purity and efficacy and standardizes the dosages. Bioidentical hormones are not FDA regulated because they come in *individualized* not standardized dosages which maximizes their effectiveness. It is important to understand however, that *all bioidentical hormone ingredients are FDA approved for use.* Bioidentical hormones are also provided by compounding pharmacies that follow the same state regulations as any other pharmacy. Added to those safety measures, the Pharmacy Compounding Accreditation Board (PCAB) applies its own set of stringent standards that compounding pharmacies must also meet.

Supporters of conjugated and synthetic hormones also like to claim that because bioidentical hormone prescriptions are formulated by hand the level of ingredients aren't consistent from one prescription to another, altering their effectiveness. They liken compounding to cooking, putting in a pinch of this and a dash of that with no real measurement of any ingredient. This is absurd. With a doctor's order, a compounding pharmacist, using industry-approved measuring instruments, is able to raise or lower the amounts of individual hormones to give a woman the ideal combination that works uniquely for her. This frees women from being locked into standardized doses that may either be too much or too little to be appropriately effective. With hormones, very small amounts make very big differences and accuracy requires flexibility in dosing.

It's also common for detractors to point out that the American Medical Association (AMA) doesn't endorse bioidentical hormones because of a lack of research. That's because nearly all research studies are paid for by the pharmaceutical corporations that want to promote their products. Even the WHI that used Premarin and Prempro was partially funded by Wyeth-Ayerst, the company that makes Premarin. Who's going to fund a national study on bioidentical hormones that can't be patented and no one can profit from?

Fortunately, we have over 50 years of women who have taken bioidentical hormones without a problem. In addition to decades of anecdotal success, two independent studies on bioidentical hormones are bearing out what we've always known.

Reassuring Results

The Early versus Late Intervention Trial with Estradiol (ELITE) study sponsored by the National Institute on Aging and performed at the Keck School of Medicine at the University of Southern California examined whether bioidentical estradiol slowed the progression of atherosclerosis in women. Test subjects without a uterus took only estradiol while those with a uterus also took bioidentical progesterone. Accumulation in the carotid artery was examined by ultrasound.

Results showed that bioidentical HT did slow the progression of atherosclerosis in women, particularly for those in the early stages of menopause. Older women who were further past menopause, while experiencing no negative effects, did not receive the same benefit.[14] These results were confirmed in follow-up studies.[15] This seems to fit with other findings that show women receive protection against cardiovascular and other diseases from HT the earlier they begin. Hormones are about timing.

The Kronos Early Estrogen Prevention Study (KEEPS) was conducted by the Kronos Longevity Research Institute in Phoenix, AZ. The goal of the double-blind, randomized, controlled study was to discover whether conjugated or bioidentical estrogen decreased the risk of heart disease in women if started within a few years after menopause. Over 720 women between the ages of 42 and 58 who were within three years of menopause were divided into three groups. The first group took oral Premarin (0.45mg/day), a dose much lower than used during the WHI (0.625mg/day). The second group took bioidentical estradiol via transdermal patch (50ug/day). Both groups were given bioidentical progesterone. The third group was placebo.

Results released showed that neither Premarin nor bioidentical estradiol had any negative effects on blood pressure. It seems probable that the benefit for the Premarin group was the result of a much lower dose than was given during the WHI as well as getting some help from the bioidentical progesterone. The majority of studies have shown Premarin *with* synthetic progestin does pose some risk of heart attack and stroke.

Premarin increased HDL (good cholesterol) and lowered LDL (bad cholesterol) but also *increased triglycerides*. Bioidentical estradiol had no positive or negative effects on cholesterol but it did improve insulin sensitivity (reduced insulin resistance). At these doses, neither Premarin nor bioidentical estradiol had any impact either way on atherosclerosis. Both relieved symptoms and increased bone density while neither group experienced any major health crisis, cancer, or cardiovascular event during the study.[16] In a new analysis of the KEEPS data [17] researchers stated, "This information should provide reassurance to women with low cardiovascular risk who are considering use of hormone treatment to reduce menopausal symptoms."[18]

It comes as no surprise that during the tests, bioidentical estradiol had zero negative effects. In addition to relieving menopause symptoms and increasing bone density it improved insulin sensitivity. This means that it's protecting women against all the diseases that are connected to insulin resistance, a benefit Premarin didn't provide. This is most certainly due to its bioidentical and easily metabolized structure. The fact that Premarin raised triglycerides is a concern and needs more study.

Honoring Life

Women have been taking both conventional and bioidentical hormones for over half a century now without a major health crisis. This is what we know for sure. Women starting HT earlier, within five years of menopause, receive the greatest benefits and disease protection while HT should never be started for the first time *after age 60*. That's when real problems occur. Women with a uterus taking estrogen *must also* take progesterone to prevent thickening of the uterine lining. Tests also repeatedly show small but viable risks for cardiovascular disease and cancer when using conventional estrogen (Premarin) especially in conjunction with synthetic progestin (Provera/Prempro). Because bioidentical hormones have shown no detrimental health effects whatsoever in testing or over the last 50 years, it's no surprise that I recommend them to my patients when needed. Besides, what could be a better replacement for your own hormones than your own hormones?

Hormones have a variety of delivery systems including capsules, sublingual pills, patches, creams, and gels. Each woman will have her preference based on how they work for her. Bioidentical progesterone must be taken orally because it's not absorbed well by transdermal methods. When you begin and how long you're on HT is between you and your doctor. My recommendation is that levels remain light, just enough to alleviate symptoms. The goal isn't to return to the energy level of your 20s. We must honor the natural progression of life while at the same time using the tools we have to give us the best quality of life at the time of life we're already in.

Chapter 18

Personal Delivery

Midwives bring simplicity and intimacy back to birthing

It might seem hard to believe but relatively recently in only 1900, 95% of all babies were born at home. In 1938, the rate had dropped to 50% and by 1955 99% of all babies were born in the hospital.[1] While hospital births seem perfectly normal to us today the truth is that women have been helping other women have babies at home for hundreds of thousands of years, and the move to medicalize the birthing process is a very recent development in human history.

Birthing Becomes Business

Prior to the second half of the 20th century, most babies were born at home with the assistance of a midwife, a woman specifically trained in the birthing process and the needs of the female body. In fact, the term midwife comes from the Old English term meaning *with woman*. As hospitals were formed and later grew into profit-based entities, the push was on to reframe childbirth as a medical procedure that required oversight instead of a natural process of the female body conducted at home.

When birthing became part of the medical business model, the experience changed drastically for both mother and child. Because childbirth became the most common procedure performed at hospitals, the profit was good but the process had to be streamlined to accommodate all expectant mothers. Unfortunately, this uniformity of process stripped away much of the attention previously paid to the spiritual and emotional needs of mother and child in favor of a sole focus on biological issues. Assuming a pregnant woman didn't have any complex health conditions, she could expect to receive the same treatment as any other woman with conveyor belt-like precision.

Today, time is money. Birthing rooms can't be occupied for too long so extended labors aren't encouraged. While most women are administered an epidural for their pain, this often slows down the dilation process. In order to speed things back up again, a woman is usually prescribed Pitocin which induces contractions that are longer, stronger, and closer together. Unfortunately, the pain is often too intense, requiring another epidural injection. This slows down the contractions which means more Pitocin and so on. Eventually, this process creates contractions that are so severe that the baby's heart and respiration rates become extremely distressed. Not long after that, the woman often finds herself being wheeled into the delivery room for an emergency C-section that was artificially induced by what were mostly unnecessary medical interventions.

Health Risks, Financial Returns

In recent years, some health professionals have begun to take note of the increasing number of healthy women with no pregnancy complications who end up having emergency C-sections after induced labor or other unnecessary medical interventions. Research from the American College of Obstetricians and Gynecologists (ACOG) has shown that the risk of needing a C-section rises sharply when labor is induced, especially if it's the first child.[2]

Unfortunately, as hospitals rush to be more competitive and serve more patients, the number of C-section births has continued to rise. Statistics from the CDC showed that between 1996 and 2007 the rate of C-section births for the U.S. rose 53% the largest increase ever recorded. In Connecticut, New Hampshire, Rhode Island, Florida, and Colorado, the increases were between 70% and 80%.[3] Today, one in every three U.S. babies (1.8 million) is born via C-section.[4]

C-section births have become so common now that most of us don't think twice when we hear a woman we know has had one, but the truth is a C-section is classified as *major surgery*. Lots of complications can occur, including hemorrhaging and blood clots for the mother or the baby requiring intensive care for various issues. Even though these risks increase with subsequent procedures,[5] C-sections are now the most common surgery performed in hospitals.[6]

In order to keep women accustomed to C-sections, they're often told that a vaginal delivery is no longer possible after the procedure. This isn't quite accurate. Additional research from the ACOG shows that 60% to 80% of women can have a successful vaginal birth after a C-section.[7] Perhaps the reason for this misdirection is that C-sections, being surgery, always cost significantly more and often twice as much as a vaginal delivery depending on the state where the child is born.[8]

Unseen Sacrifices

This isn't to say that C-sections are bad. They save lives when they're absolutely necessary. The real issue is why and how they become "necessary" for so many otherwise healthy women who choose a hospital birth.

Another concern with C-sections is that because the baby does not travel through the birth canal, a final surge of the hormone oxytocin isn't triggered. Oxytocin is the "love" hormone that generates intense feelings of euphoria, overwhelm, and bonding between mother and child. Oxytocin is also generated on a much smaller scale during breastfeeding. Because this big hormone rush that normally sets bonding patterns in place doesn't happen during a C-section, feelings of attachment to the baby can be somewhat lessened.

Studies of MRI brain scans from Yale University have shown some C-section mothers to be lacking in attachment to their babies or less sensitive to their baby's upset than mothers who gave birth vaginally.[9] Oftentimes monkeys given C-sections will ignore their babies. Oxytocin also works synergistically with serotonin as a mood elevator which might explain why C-section mothers experience postpartum depression more often, but additional research needs to be done in this regard.

In a vaginal birth, the baby becomes covered in the mucosal lining of the birth canal with much of it entering its nose, mouth, and ears. This lining is populated with billions of various strains of probiotics that once ingested serve as the first inoculation of the baby's gut, establishing the primary culture of what will become its intestinal flora and immune system. In a C-section, this vital inoculation doesn't happen, leaving the baby's immunity compromised and struggling to catch up later in life.

Priorities & Process

As hospital birthing continues to become more mechanized, increasing numbers of women are looking to midwives and home birth to bring a sense of personalization, peace, and less trauma back to what is essentially a sacred process for themselves and their babies. In general, a midwife remains with an expectant mother throughout her entire pregnancy. This includes monitoring her physical and emotional wellbeing, providing individualized education, counseling, prenatal care, gynecological exams, hands-on assistance during labor, delivery, and postpartum support, lactation consultation, and providing referrals for additional obstetric care. A midwife may practice independently or in association with a doctor's office.

A woman can also use a midwife in addition to the care she's already receiving from her OBGYN whether she chooses of have a home birth or not. Midwives are qualified to deliver babies at home, in the hospital, or at separate birthing centers. Midwifery is currently overseen by the American College of Nurse Midwives (ACNM), Midwives Alliance of North America (MANA), North American Registry of Midwives (NARM) and the Midwifery Education Accreditation Council along with the support group Citizens for Midwifery.

At present, there are four types of midwife designations. **Certified Nurse Midwives** (CNM) hold either a Bachelor's or Master's Degree in Nursing and have passed a national certification exam administered by the ACNM, earning them a state license to practice. **Certified Midwives** (CM) also receive their certification from the ACNM but hold degrees in areas other than nursing. **Certified Professional Midwives** (CPM) are trained midwives who have been certified through NARM. The credential requires re-certification every three years. **Direct Entry Midwives** (DEM) may or may not hold a college degree but have trained in apprenticeship and other instructional programs which include attending home births and those at birthing centers.

Whether you are interested in becoming a midwife or using a midwife's services, it's very important to first find out which certifications your state recognizes. You can do this by reaching out to your state midwifery organization through contact information provided by Citizens for Midwifery. Be sure your midwife is certified with ample experience. Ask lots of questions and always check references with previous mothers they have served. Interview potential midwives in person. A successful experience depends equally on how your personalities and philosophies match up as much as credentials. Additional information can be obtained from contacting ACNM and NARM, as well.

Impressive Outcomes

Even though midwives are thoroughly trained and professionally certified, modern society's exclusive familiarity with hospital birth might leave some people doubting the safety of birthing at home. Hospital birthing *has* to be safer because well, it's in the hospital. Right? Actually, the world was populated long before hospitals, but let's look at some statistics.

In 2023, the U.S. ranked 174th out of 227 countries with an infant mortality rate of 5.1 deaths per 1,000 live births, far behind nearly every other western industrialized nation. [10] Because 99% of all births today take place in hospitals, it's clear these mortality rates can't be coming from babies born at home.

On the contrary, a study published by the *British Medical Journal* following more than 5,000 expectant mothers in North America who chose a home birth with a certified nurse midwife showed they required substantially less of almost every medical intervention, including epidurals, episiotomy, forceps, vacuum extraction, and C-section, and experienced virtually no neonatal or intrapartum mortality.[11]

The NARM website provides quite a few research studies published by internationally recognized medical journals that consistently confirm the high rate of safety and positive outcomes for low-risk women birthing at home with the assistance of a midwife. One study published in the *Journal of Midwifery and Women's Health* stated that home births rose 41% in the U.S. between 2004 and 2010. It examined outcomes of nearly 17,000 women who planned to give birth at home between 2004 and 2009.

Of that total, 89.1% had a successful home birth. The majority of the women who had to be transferred to the hospital arrived for "failure to progress" with only 4.5% of the total sample requiring Pitocin to induce labor and/or an epidural. A vaginal birth was accomplished by 93.6% and assisted vaginal birth by 1.2% while just 5.2% had a C-section, a far cry from the national C-section average of 33%. Of the 1,054 women in the sample who attempted a vaginal birth after a previous C-section, 87% were successful. Postpartum hospital transfers for mother and child were just 1.5% and 0.9% respectively. Most of the babies (86%) were exclusively breastfeeding by 6 weeks of age. The intrapartum, early neonatal, and late neonatal mortality rates were 1.3, 0.41 and 0.35 per 1,000. That's significantly lower than the U.S. average of 5.1 per 1,000. The researchers acknowledge that, "Low-risk women in this cohort experienced high rates of physiologic [vaginal] birth and low rates of intervention without an increase in adverse outcomes."[12]

A study from the National Center for Health Statistics published in the *Journal of Epidemiology and Community Health* followed all single vaginal births in the U.S. in 1991 attended by either a physician or certified nurse midwife (CNM). It stated that mortality rates in the births overseen by midwives showed "excellent outcomes." In fact, the risk of infant death was 19% lower for births assisted by a CNM than they were for births conducted by physicians. The risk of neonatal mortality (infant death in the first 28 days after birth) was 33% lower with a CNM than with a doctor while the risk for low birth weight was 31% lower.[13]

Exceeding Standard Practice

Naturally, these kinds of successful numbers have left some doctors looking down on midwives, feeling competitive and insecure. At times, this has been known to create a rift between the two groups, especially in rare cases where a woman has a very long labor or an unforeseen complication that requires a midwife to accompany the mother to the hospital. Her reception from the doctor can be professional but tense. Of course, none of this helps the expectant mother who should be the sole focus of the situation and not professional egos. She's already disappointed that she couldn't birth at home and doesn't need an uncompassionate doctor making her feel like she's inconveniencing his schedule.

It's because doctors don't see the vast majority of births that happen smoothly and uneventfully at home but only the rare case that needs hospital intervention, that they have a wild misperception of professional midwives. The goal should be to work collaboratively with midwives to provide the expectant mother with the highest quality of care based on where, how, and with whom she chooses to have her baby. If home birth plans change, then a doctor should be fully committed to continuing to provide, as much as possible, the same kind of birthing experience the mother would have had at home with only the technological interventions that are absolutely necessary while working alongside the midwife.

Unfortunately, the American Medical Association (AMA) wasn't keen on collaboration when they released an official statement saying, "...the safest setting for labor, delivery, and the immediate postpartum period is in a hospital or birthing center within a hospital."[14] It's interesting that the AMA didn't mention midwives in their statement, especially since midwives can accompany women to the hospital who have chosen them to oversee their hospital birth, many of whom have practice privileges in hospitals.

Fortunately, most OBGYNs know and respect their patients. They're more than willing to work with a midwife throughout a woman's pregnancy and be ready to meet them at the hospital when the time comes if need be. What all doctors need to understand is that they were educated in a system that's very reductionist and breaks the human body down into separate, impersonal, mechanical parts with a one-size-fits-all approach to care, especially for childbirth. Melissa Cheyney, lead researcher on the study of 17,000 home births said, "The U.S. has a limited idea of what it means to have a positive outcome at the end of a delivery. Basically, it just means that everyone is alive."[15]

What many doctors weren't taught to recognize was how a woman interacts synergistically with her unborn baby and even her own body during the pregnancy and birth process. Surely women deserve more from the healthcare system than simple relief that nothing went wrong during their delivery. They deserve the kind of experience that connects them with their body in a way like no other and reunites them with the profound sacredness of what it means to bring another human being into this world, surely a woman's greatest gift. With a little more focus on personalization instead of profit we can provide that kind of experience for every woman. Even within an imperfect health system we can work together to give each mother and child what they deserve, a truly personal delivery.

Chapter 19

Early Detection Disaster

How prostate cancer screening failed men

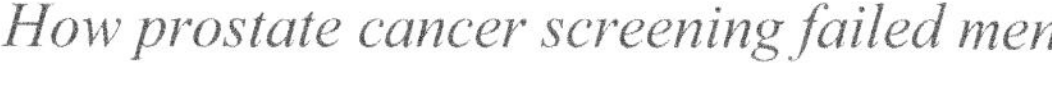

Today, the fight against cancer has largely become a race game for early detection and treatment. Unfortunately, we're finding that the early detection screening methods we once held up as the gold standard are seriously flawed and, in some cases, entirely inaccurate. This is exactly the situation with the prostate specific antigen (PSA), the test that since 1994 has been the premier screening method for prostate cancer. Now, more than three decades of rushing into treatment is revealing how the lives of tens of millions of men were ruined, fortunes were created, and a healthcare disaster exploded.

Runaway Mistake

In 1970, Dr. Richard J. Albin, PhD discovered an antigen (protein) that was specific to prostate cancer that could be used in diagnosing the condition. Unfortunately, what he found, the prostate specific antigen (PSA) was present in *both* the benign (normal) and malignant prostate. There was no way to tell if a man had prostate cancer using the PSA but with some additional analysis it was helpful for tracking the prostate for *a recurrence of cancer* but only *after* it had already been diagnosed and treated. As an initial diagnostic tool for prostate cancer, the PSA test was useless.

In 1986, the FDA approved the PSA test as a tool to track the *recurrence* of prostate cancer. Biotech executives weren't happy because they wanted the PSA approved for cancer detection. Not only would that have meant a bigger market and higher profits, but it also would have boosted development in immunotherapy drugs.

Although only one lab was approved to produce PSA test kits, several other labs started doing so and soon the market was flooded with off-label test kits being used to diagnose prostate cancer. The misuse was so widespread that the FDA relented and approved the PSA test for prostate cancer detection in 1994, recommending all men be tested beginning at age 50.

In the end, habitual misuse and profit-hungry corporations that wanted to sell a prostate cancer prevention scam won. It was tens of millions of American men who lost. The PSA test had no cutoff for detecting cancer. Some men with a PSA level as low as 0.5ng/mL actually had prostate cancer while those with a level as high as 11ng/mL didn't. The test didn't mean anything and yet men testing as low as 4ng/mL were immediately sent for a biopsy. Since the test couldn't decipher between benign or malignant cells, if there was any sign of cancer men were rushed into harmful treatments like radiation, chemotherapy, and prostate removal. As a result, tens of millions of men were left with urinary incontinence, impotence, hormonal imbalance and the intense depression that comes with such abrupt and severe biological changes.

In a 2010 op-ed article in the *New York Times* titled, *The Great Prostate Mistake*, Dr. Albin revealed the FDA based their 1994 approval of the PSA test on research that showed it could detect prostate cancer in just 3.8% of cases.[1] In his book, *The Great Prostate Hoax: How big medicine hijacked the PSA test and caused a public health disaster*, Dr. Albin lamented, "With the 78% false positive rate and being wrong 80% of the time, I don't know how the test was approved."[2]

Considering the fact that the PSA is wrong 80% of the time and that approximately 30 million men each year for the last 30 years had the test, the number of men who have had their lives ruined by the rush to treatment is staggering.[3] Today, researchers are finally admitting PSA screening doesn't reduce death rates in men 55 and older.[4] The tragic truth is that with very rare exceptions, prostate cancer is extremely slow-growing. In fact, it's so slow that the vast majority of those men from decades ago could have lived full, happy lives and never died of prostate cancer. Most men don't.

Turning the Tide

While the news media was reluctant to report on the limitations of the PSA test and how the rush into drastic treatment was ruining men's health, influential healthcare agencies were changing their minds about the test and its efficacy. The United States Preventative Services Task Force stated that there was "convincing evidence that a substantial percentage of men who have asymptomatic cancer detected by PSA screening have a tumor that either will not progress or will progress so slowly that it would have remained asymptomatic for the man's lifetime" and that the "over-diagnosis" from prostate cancer screening using the PSA test was as high as 50%. As such, it concluded that "...the USPSTF now recommends against PSA-based screening for prostate cancer in all age groups."[5]

After that announcement, a survey of Massachusetts doctors found 80% said the PSA test "offered more harm than benefit" and the American Cancer Society urged "more caution" when pursuing PSA screening. [6] The Prostate Cancer Foundation, National Cancer Institute, and American Urological Association all recommended that men make an informed decision with their doctor before having a PSA test. Stricter guidelines were provided only for those men who were either African American because they have a higher rate of prostate cancer than other men and/or those who had a family history of cancer.

The most logical recommendation now is to watch and wait while discussing treatment options with your doctor. This is the wisest and most humane approach, especially since American men have only a 12.5% chance of developing prostate cancer during their lifetime and just a 3% chance of actually dying from it.[7] Don't rush into treatment or make any rash decisions.

Prostate Basics

The prostate gland is about the size of a walnut and located on the underside of the bladder between it and the penis, just in front of the rectum. It's a complex, spongy structure made up of tiny sacs from which fluid is secreted to protect the sperm.

The urethra runs from the bladder through the center of the prostate and into the penis to allow urine to flow out of the body.

During ejaculation, the prostate squeezes this fluid into the urethra where it's expelled with sperm as semen. The vas deferens bring sperm from the testes to the seminal vesicles that connect to the prostate from behind which also contribute fluid to the ejaculate.

As men age, the prostate can lose some of its suppleness. This limits its ability to vigorously contract and fully expel all its fluids. The result is a retrograde ejaculation where men either don't release completely or have a muted orgasm.

When the prostate cannot fully empty, residual fluid builds up and like the deposits in the bottom of a drinking glass, they crystalize and calcify over time. It's this calcification that causes the prostate to become progressively more rigid by limiting its ability to fully contract. The stagnant fluid and its deposits also invite infection.

Problems & Priorities

The standard test for prostate health is the digital rectal exam during which the physician inserts a lubricated, gloved finger into the rectum to detect enlargement, potentially cancerous lumps, nodules, or tenderness that might suggest prostatitis. During this procedure, massaging of the prostate may occur to help it release fluid through the penis. In this way, it can be tested along with a urine sample. White blood cells and pathogens present in the samples reveal an infection.

Prostatitis, the most common prostate illness in men, occurs when the prostate becomes infected by bacteria, viruses, mycoplasma, or other nonbacterial agents. If prostatitis is untreated and becomes chronic, the inflammation from the infection will cause the prostate to enlarge, creating burning sensations during urination. As the prostate continues to swell, it increasingly constricts the urethra, narrowing the pathway through which urine can pass out of the body, making urination slow and difficult. This enlargement of the prostate is known as benign prostatic hypertrophy (BPH).

Alpha blockers can relax the muscles around the urethra in men with an enlarged prostate, allowing urine to flow more freely. 5-alpha-reductase inhibitors can reduce levels of dihydrotestosterone (DHT) which run high when the prostate is enlarged. DHT is the hormone linked to hair loss. Its levels increase as men age. Lowering

DHT levels can help shrink the prostate.

At the same time, antibiotics may be prescribed for a prostate infection, but the challenge is that very few of the medications to which prostate pathogens are sensitive are able to pass through the plasma-prostate barrier and into the prostatic fluid. Because of this, antibiotics-only therapy works in just one out of three cases.[8]

Unchecked prostate inflammation from BPH often leads to an eventual diagnosis of prostate cancer, particularly because inflammation is a primary factor in the development of all cancers. If cancer is present, a prostate ultrasound can be performed by inserting an ultrasound probe into the rectum and is usually conducted in conjunction with a biopsy.

Although prostate cancer is typically a slow-growing cancer which men rarely die from, particularly when diagnosed late in life, a swollen, rigid, and inflamed prostate negatively impacts a man's quality of life in many ways. Because of this, prostate health should be his number one priority moving into middle age.

Rejection Remembered

As with other illnesses, prostate problems can have a psycho-spiritual component. Problems in the urogenital organs always reflect unresolved emotional issues connected with sex, relationships, and for men beliefs about masculinity.

This was the case with Alan, the owner of a software development company. He had been battling prostate hypertrophy for nearly a decade. His prostate had become so large that it was severely hardened and pushing against the bladder. This reduced the bladder's volume capacity and left him with the constant sensation of having to urinate. When he did go to the bathroom, the prostate intrusion into his bladder didn't allow him to empty completely. All the doctors he had previously seen recommended surgery.

I treated Alan for several weeks and gave him some pyscho-spiritual exercises to do. Each time I asked him about past relationship difficulties, his answers were limited and nonchalant.

His treatment involved receiving an injection of homeopathics into his perineum while I performed a manual manipulation of the prostate. One day, I decided to ask him questions regarding his past relationships during the procedure. After several uninformative responses, I asked if he had ever felt rejected by a woman. Perhaps it was the word rejected that sparked his response, but Alan answered with more emotion than I had ever heard from him.

He began telling me the story of how, as a volunteer, he had fallen head over heels in love with a summer camp counselor more than 30 years earlier. After a terrific summer experience, the woman decided to go off with one of the other counselors, reducing him to just a summer fling. The experience left him feeling horribly rejected and would color his relationship activity for the next several years.

Before Alan even finished telling me the story, I knew his prostate was receding. The change was dramatic, but I said nothing. Within days he called me reporting incredible improvements. His discomfort and frequent urination were gone as were his sexual performance problems. He was even able to completely empty his bladder.

I asked him to come in and take a PSA test. When his results came back, I was stunned. His PSA went from 9.2 to 3.8. I asked him to abstain from all sexual activity so I could test him again one week later to confirm the results. They were the same. His symptoms have never returned.

Prostate Massage

Once prostatitis reaches the chronic stage, it's extremely difficult to eradicate as relapses are common. The best approach for prostatitis is a preventative prostate massage two to four times per year after age 50. The primary goal of a prostate massage is to drain the residual fluid to prevent hardened deposits from forming and providing an environment hospitable to microbes. Prostate massage can also help ease tension around nerve endings behind the prostate in the levator ani muscle in a form of myofascial release to relieve pain.

A prostate massage is similar to a digital rectal exam. During the procedure, the physician inserts a lubricated, gloved finger into the rectum and gently massages the prostate. Once the prostate is properly relaxed and primed, a probe is inserted to make contact with it. At that time, the physician guides the patient through a pattern of deep breathing, holding, and muscle contractions as the probe lightly oscillates and vibrates against the prostate in order to break up calcified deposits. After a few minutes an additional massage of the prostate is performed known as "milking" the prostate in order to encourage fluid and particles to be expelled through the penis.

Prostate massage is not new. Up until the 1960s when certain drugs became available, it was the primary treatment for prostatitis. Studies show that the most effective treatment for prostatitis is a dual approach that includes both antibiotics and prostate massage.[9] A study from the Philippines showed that patients with chronic prostatitis receiving antibiotics and prostate massage three times a week for 12 weeks reported significant decreases in symptom severity of greater than 60% that lasted into the two-year follow-up.[10]

Purging as Prevention

Adding more evidence to the importance of regularly purging the prostate are two recent long-term, large-scale studies. It's always been known anecdotally that men who ejaculate more regularly have lower rates of prostate cancer. Now an eighteen-year study following 30,000 men has confirmed it scientifically. The study, which examined men between ages 46 and 81, found that those who ejaculated 21 or more times per month had a 33% less chance of developing prostate cancer than men who reported ejaculating between four and seven times per month.[11]

An Australian study following 2,300 men came to the same conclusion. Men who averaged 4.6 to 7 ejaculations per week were 36% less likely to develop prostate cancer by age 70 than men who ejaculated an average of 2.3 times per week.[12]

While it's now clear that frequent and full release of the prostate is essential for the prevention of prostate cancer, a study published in *European Urology* explored whether gene expression patterns varied according to frequency of ejaculation. Analyzing 20,254 genes in 157 men who developed prostate cancer from the earlier eighteen-year study, researchers found 409 genes and six pathways significantly associated with ejaculation frequency. They stated in their findings that less frequent ejaculation can trigger genetic changes that lead to cancer. The researchers stated, "These results suggest that ejaculation affects the expression of genes in the normal prostate tissue. The identified genes and pathways provide potential biological links between [ejaculation frequency] and prostate tumorigenesis."[13]

The time to think about a prostate massage is before prostatitis develops and you really do need one. To mitigate nervousness, it might help to think about clearing out your old prostatic fluid the same way you change the oil in your car because that's basically what you're doing. They both need to be done about every three months anyway.

The results in my patients who have regular prostate massage are often dramatic. Conditions like erectile dysfunction, premature ejaculation, burning during urination, and chronic pelvic pain all significantly improve or resolve completely. I had a patient whose prostate was so swollen and painful that he couldn't sit down. When his pain disappeared, he was overjoyed.

The key for men to maintaining health as they age is to take care of the prostate. To do this, they must put the necessary time and prevention into regular prostate massage after age 50. Forget about self-consciousness. This is about self-care and making sure the rest of your life is the best of your life. With a bit of awareness and the right preventative health choices, men can give themselves the best chance of avoiding everything from prostatitis to prostate cancer, enjoying optimal function and sexual performance well into later life.

Chapter 20

Keeping the Edge

Maintaining healthy testosterone levels for men

When most of us think of testosterone, we think of it in terms of sex drive. While testosterone is crucial for a healthy libido even in women, in men it's absolutely vital for mental and physical health by supporting things like proper bone density, cardiovascular health, better sleep, lean muscle growth, sense of wellbeing, attention, memory, motivation, ambition, and assertiveness.

Because testosterone serves so many important functions in a man's body, it's important that he understands how to naturally keep his levels high in order to remain healthier longer as he moves into middle age and beyond. While bioidentical testosterone replacement is always an option after a man enters his 60s, there is much he can do earlier in life to maximize his own testosterone production so that replacement therapy isn't necessary.

What's Normal?

A man's testosterone production peaks sometime between his late teens and early 20s then starts to gradually decline starting at age 30. A male infant starts life with serum testosterone levels less than 30 nanograms per deciliter (ng/dl). Teens 14 to 15 average 8 to 53 ng/dl, while young men 16 to 19 see levels between 200 and 970 ng/dl. By their 20s or early 30s, men show testosterone levels ranging from 270 to 1,080 ng/dl. Between ages 40 and 59, levels drop to between 350 and 890 ng/dl while after age 60 levels run from 350 to 720 ng/dl.

As you can see, these normal ranges are extremely broad. The most important point to understand from this is that there is no "normal" level of testosterone for men, only the level that's normal for you. All men are different and as such, have wildly varying levels of testosterone between them. What matters is how a man feels and functions at a certain level. One 40-year-old man may have lots of energy and a healthy sex drive at 510 ng/dl when another man the same age feels lethargic and depressed at 725 ng/dl. While both men are in the "normal" range for their age, it's clear the second man's testosterone is not at his personal normal level.

Far too many men suffering from the effects of age-related low testosterone are told by their doctors that their levels are "in the normal range" so hormones couldn't be the cause of the problems they're experiencing. Either their symptoms end up getting treated with multiple medications or they're handed a prescription for an antidepressant and sent home.

In order for a man to know exactly what his normal testosterone level is without any guesswork, he needs to have it checked while he's still in his 20s during the prime of his life, feeling vibrant and healthy. Knowing that number will give a doctor an important baseline to work from should testosterone replacement therapy (TRT) become an issue for the man later in life. The idea isn't to give a 65-year-old man the testosterone levels he had at 25, but the number will show doctors whether he needs to be on the high or low end of his current age-related range or somewhere in between. Hormone replacement requires a lot of fine tuning in each patient, and having a baseline from earlier in life takes most of the guesswork out of the process.

Half the Man

Symptoms of low testosterone include low libido, difficulty with erections, low energy, fatigue, lethargy, depression, lack of sense of wellbeing, moodiness, trouble with memory, lack of focus or motivation, difficulty concentrating, loss of muscle mass, unexplained weight gain, decreased bone mass, low semen volume, and anemia. According to the American Urological Association, two out of 10 men over 60 experience low testosterone levels. After age 70, it's 3 in 10.[1]

While aged-related low testosterone for senior men is understandable, new research is raising concern as it reveals a significant drop in testosterone levels for younger men. Perhaps this is why a recent report in the *Journal of the American Medical Association* found that TRT among American men has doubled since 2010.[2] In fact, studies show that men's testosterone levels have been declining for decades and that men today have less testosterone than men of the same age a generation ago. Hormonally speaking, men today are half the men their fathers and grandfathers used to be.

A study published in *The Journal of Clinical Endocrinology and Metabolism* found what it called a "substantial" drop in testosterone levels for U.S. men since the 1980s with average levels declining at 1% per year. This means that in 2002 a man age 65 had a testosterone level 15% lower than a man age 65 in 1987. Results also indicated that the greater portion of the male population in 2002 had below-normal testosterone levels than men of the same age in 1987.[3] A Danish study found similar results of a 14% drop when comparing the testosterone levels of men born in the 1960s versus the 1920s. This was accompanied by a 26% decline in sex hormone-binding globulin (SHBG) during the same time period. Researchers called the results "a little frightening."[4]

Adding to the alarm, European studies have shown sperm counts are also declining among young men which coincides with a decrease in musculoskeletal strength.[5] This was reflected in a 2016 study that showed the average man age 20 to 34 could only exert 98 lbs. of right-hand grip strength when compared to 117 lbs. from men the same age in 1985.[6] Of course, grip strength isn't indicative of overall fitness but research has found it to be a significant predictor of all-cause mortality, particularly from cardiovascular conditions.[7]

Environmental Offenders

Researchers have been puzzled as to what is causing the downward trend in testosterone and sperm counts which is happening predominantly in men in the western world. While excess body fat does decrease testosterone and increase estrogen, the testosterone decline has persisted in studies even after researchers controlled for obesity and other variables.

Chemicals

Recently, more suspicion has been directed toward environmental toxins as the cause. These include fungicides, herbicides, and pesticides heavily sprayed on crops that all include chemicals classified as xeno-estrogens or compounds that mimic estrogen and have estrogenic effects inside the body. Most personal care products like lotions, shampoos, deodorants, and colognes contain xeno-estrogens in the form of phthalates and parabens. Any chemical ingredient that includes either of these title extensions is an endocrine disruptor. The same holds true for all household cleaning products and air fresheners. Phthalates are most often hidden in these products under the generically listed “fragrance.” In fact, almost all artificial fragrance is the result of phthalates that we breathe in. Bisphenol A, a chemical that provides flexibility for plastics, also has estrogenic properties and has been known to leach into liquids contained in plastic bottles. Prior to the 1990s, most liquid food products were contained in glass. Now, everything from soda to mayonnaise comes in a plastic bottle or container.

Soy

Soy is another serious contributor to low testosterone because of the phytoestrogens (plant-based estrogens) also known as isoflavones that it contains. Isoflavones can latch onto cellular hormone receptors and reduce the body’s natural hormone production or prevent us from utilizing our own hormones. In fact, isoflavones are so similar in structure to human estrogen that bioidentical estrogen used in hormone replacement therapy for women is made from soy.

Birth control pills are mostly estrogen and trick a woman’s body into thinking it’s already pregnant because estrogen levels rise during pregnancy. Soy isoflavones work exactly the same way and have been proven to cause complete infertility in sheep, cows,[8] and rodents.[9] In comparison, the Swiss Health Service stated that 100 g of isoflavones per day contains the same level of estrogen as a birth control pill.[10]

In a man's body, soy has a significant detrimental effect on fertility. A study from Harvard University published in *Human Reproduction* found that men who consumed just ½ serving of soy per day in the form of foods like tofu, soy ice cream, miso soup, or energy bars had 41 million fewer sperm per milliliter than men who did not consume soy.[11] That's the profound effect after consuming the equivalent of just one cup of soy milk *every other day*. Normal sperm counts range between 80 million and 120 million sperm per milliliter. Unless a man is at the very high end of this range, losing 41 million sperm per milliliter would drop him well below normal and risk infertility.

Both Russian and Italian research has shown that rats fed genetically modified (GMO) soy experience damage to their sperm, and the DNA in their offspring exhibits altered function. In addition, the testicles experience extreme discoloration.[12] Over 90% of all soy grown in the U.S. is GMO.[13]

Cell Phone Radiation

Electromagnetic radiation is also well-known to damage reproductive organs. Studies have shown that men who carried cell phones in their pants pocket experienced a significant decrease in sperm production and sperm motility with an increase in sperm cell deformity.[14] Other research has shown that men who wore their cell phones on a belt clip and used it extensively over a five-day period had a 19% decrease in high sperm motility[15] with a corresponding decrease in sperm count.[16] Studies have been confirming the detrimental effect of cell phone radiation on sperm since 2002.[17]

Illicit, Prescription, and Over-the-Counter Drugs

Illicit, prescribed, and over-the-counter drugs can reduce testosterone and sperm counts. Antihistamines and drugs for acid reflux often contain Cimetidine which blocks testosterone synthesis.[18] Ketoconazole, an ingredient found in drugs for dermatitis, athlete's foot, and dandruff also interrupts testosterone production.[19] Because all sex hormones are synthesized from cholesterol, statins (cholesterol lowering drugs) decrease testosterone levels.[20] It has long been known that recreational drugs, especially marijuana, not only reduce sperm counts and testosterone[21] but cause testicular shrinkage.[22]

Role Reversal

In the ongoing attempt to solve the strangely universal decrease in testosterone and sperm counts across the western world, some have gone so far as to offer an epigenetic explanation. Today, young men mostly work in offices with no demand for real physical labor. Therefore, their bodies have adapted to not be as strong as previous generations of men.

At the same time, as women's salaries continued to increase, we saw the rise of the stay-at-home dad who was bathing babies and changing diapers. When women moved into the boardroom, men increasingly moved into the classroom and examining room as teachers and nurses, traditionally female dominated occupations.

While one might celebrate this role reversal as a political victory, men's biology is experiencing this unusual trend in an entirely different way. The body responds to how we feel, particularly when behaving in certain ways or performing specific activities. As our feelings change, our biochemistry changes in thousands of ways moment to moment that have real biological effects. For example, one study from the Philippines showed that men who took care of their children at least three hours per day had 20% less testosterone than men who did not.[23]

This raises the question, regardless of how politically incorrect it may seem, as to whether it is healthy for men to be involved in the everyday nurturing care of children which for 99% of human history has been the realm of women. This isn't to say that men shouldn't be involved in the lives of their children through playing with or teaching them the important aspects of life. Research consistently shows a strong relationship with the father is crucial for a child to grow up well-adjusted.[24] The main point revolves around exactly what kinds of interaction that relationship should include and whether men should really be involved in diapering, toileting, soothing, feeding, bathing, and participating in other nurturing activities of their children. As we discussed in a previous chapter on sexual energy, these kinds of activities will keep a man inhabiting his feminine energy most of the time which isn't good for men or keeping an intimate relationship with a wife or partner sexually polarized. This is an area that deserves more research.

Pumping It Up

What can men do to support testosterone production as they age? A healthy testosterone level means better health overall. Fortunately, there are several things men can do before they resort to testosterone replacement therapy (TRT) and in many cases make it unnecessary.

Eat saturated animal fat and cholesterol

Fat and cholesterol are not the enemies when it comes to heart disease or any disease; it's sugar, simple carbohydrates, and polyunsaturated fats (processed seed oils) like vegetable oil, soybean oil, canola oil, and others. Since the 1950s, the anti-animal fat campaign has been driven by corporate food manufacturers who wanted people to purchase their processed seed oils instead of lard, tallow, and other natural fats. Even so, over 70 years of research exists that conclusively shows animal fat and cholesterol are essential for human health while the high inflammation caused by consuming processed seed oils creates heart disease and other illnesses.

One of the oldest and largest studies that is still going on today is the Framingham Heart Study that started in 1948 and includes 15,000 people. Results consistently show that *declining* cholesterol levels in people over 50 result in proportional *increases* in death from cardiovascular disease as well as other chronic diseases. In fact, some of the first data showed that for every 1 mg/dL decrease in cholesterol, participants experienced a 14% increase in death from cardiovascular disease and an 11% increase in death from other chronic diseases. The results were so consistent that researchers stated in 1992:

> In Framingham, Mass., the more saturated fat one ate, the more cholesterol one ate, the more calories one ate, the lower the person's serum cholesterol…We found that the people who ate the most cholesterol, ate the most saturated fat, ate the most calories, weighed the least and were the most physically active."[25]

A recent review of the decades of research studies involving the alleged connection between saturated animal fat and heart disease found that:

- The large, corporate-sponsored clinical trials linking saturated fats to heart disease were flawed and *do not* provide scientific support for the connection.
- The most rigorous studies on saturated fats, showing they *did not* cause heart disease, were suppressed or ignored.
- The current 10% cap on saturated fat intake by the U.S. Dietary Guidelines for Americans is not supported by the preponderance of evidence.

The reviewers acknowledged the "fundamental inadequacy of the evidence to support the idea that saturated fats cause heart disease" and that the resistance to the real data within the medical and corporate sectors arose out of "longstanding biases" and "vested interests." They concluded, "Until the recent science on saturated fats is incorporated into the U.S. Dietary Guidelines, the policy on this topic *cannot be seen as evidence-based.*"[26]

Because nearly all of this data has been suppressed and the relentless campaign to promote seed oils as "heart healthy" has gone on for nearly three generations, it can be difficult for some people to accept the reality that saturated animal fat is good for our health. While it isn't the scope of this book to go into the details of that issue, I would recommend *The Great Cholesterol Con* by Dr. Malcolm Kendrick for additional reading. For now, let's talk about cholesterol and hormones.

Cholesterol is the precursor for the master hormone pregnenolone from which all sex hormones, including testosterone, are made. Not one hormone in the body could be made without cholesterol.[27] Researchers found that testosterone levels fell 12% after a group of men ages 50 to 60 switched from their usual high fat/low fiber diet to one that was high in fiber but low in fat.[28]

Other evidence has shown that when men cut saturated fat by as little as 15% in their diet it results in "significant" declines in serum testosterone, free testosterone, and 4-androstenedione, a vital hormone for testosterone synthesis.[29] For optimal testosterone production, it's best to aim for getting at least 50% of your daily calories from saturated fat in the form of foods like organic red meat that's well-marbled with fat, dark meat chicken, butter, avocados, coconut oil, wild caught fatty fish like sockeye salmon, lamb, and egg yolks. Testosterone is also fat-soluble, so it needs saturated fat to be utilized by the body.

It's also important to note that cholesterol is what strengthens the cell membrane of all one trillion cells of the body and gives them their integrity. The brain is 60% saturated fat and craves cholesterol which is why high cholesterol levels have been shown to improve learning and memory[30] and help prevent dementia as we age.[31]

Eat estrogen-blocking foods

Vegetables like broccoli, cauliflower, Brussels sprouts, bok choy, kale, collard greens, turnips, and rutabagas contain high levels of phytochemicals that have been shown to block estrogen production and metabolism.[32] The skin of red grapes contains resveratrol, and grape seed extract contains high levels of proanthocyanidin both of which have been shown to suppress aromatase, an enzyme that's central to estrogen production.[33]

Eliminate sugar and processed carbs

Sugar and processed carbs which turn into sugar (glucose) rapidly in the body raise insulin and cortisol levels which are natural antagonists to testosterone production. In one study, after men consumed 75 g of sugar, about the same amount in a bottle of soda, within an hour their serum testosterone levels fell by 25% and remained low for at least two hours. This caused 15% of the men to fall into the hypogonadal range where doctors declare a man's testicles to have failed.[34]

Avoid soy

This means soy in all its forms not just tofu. The tricky part is that soy is an ingredient in most processed foods usually as soybean oil or soy lecithin. Soybean oil is found abundantly in cookies, snack cakes, crackers, bread, peanut butter, and more. It also forms the base of almost all commercial salad dressings, mayonnaise, sauces, and condiments. Soy lecithin is a thickening agent added to things like pudding and thousands of other products. Always read ingredient labels. If lecithin is listed without specifying that it's from sunflower seeds or another source, it's from soy.

Work out hard and fast

Exercise, especially resistance training, is the original and best testosterone booster. Men experience a sharp increase in both testosterone and human growth hormone (HGH) after lifting weights, and the boost is even greater when the rest time between sets is limited to one minute.[35] Studies show heavy resistance training increases HGH in men by 200% to 700%.[36]

High intensity interval training (HIIT) alternates brief moments of strenuous exercise with intervals of rest. An example might be sprinting for 30 seconds then walking until you catch your breath, then sprinting for 30 seconds again over a period of 15 to 20 minutes. Another might be sprint for 60 seconds, walk for 30 seconds, pushups for 60 seconds, then walk for 30 seconds, and so on. One study found that HIIT runners alternating sprinting and walking experienced an increase in free testosterone five times higher than a group that ran at a steady pace.[37] Other research has found that a single 30-second sprint raises HGH by 450%[38] and that short bursts of intense training as with HIIT keep HGH secretion high for up to 24 hours.[39]

Adopt better body language

How we use our bodies affects how we feel which generates emotions that change our biochemistry. A joint study between

Columbia University and Harvard University found that expansive and confident poses like reclining in a chair with feet on a desk and arms behind the head or leaning over from behind a desk as if to explain something to someone actually raised testosterone levels as opposed to crossing arms in front of oneself or sitting in a chair with hands in the lap which decreased levels.[40] The body is listening, so walk more confidently, adopt a firmer handshake, or a take a broader stance, and your hormones will follow how you feel.

Keep tech gadgets away from the groin

Don't put your cell phone in your pocket or clip it to your belt. Carry it in a briefcase, backpack, or even in your hand. Just keep it away from the groin area. Never put your laptop directly on your lap. Look for an alternate flat surface even if it's an empty chair next to you at the airport.

Purge parabens and phthalates

Check all the ingredient labels of your personal care products like lotion, shaving cream, toothpaste, shampoo, and deodorant for anything that includes the extensions phthalate[41] or paraben[42] such as butylparaben. These chemicals have estrogenic effects on the body. Get rid of any offending products and find better alternatives. Do the same for all cleaning products and air fresheners.

Check your medications

If you're taking any kind of medication, read the entire insert that comes with it for hormonal side effects. This goes for over-the-counter medications, too. Research them online. If you find they disrupt hormones, ask your doctor to prescribe something else.

Lose weight

Being overweight is one of the most common causes of low testosterone in men of all ages. This is because testosterone gets converted into estrogen in fat tissue and the more fat there is the faster and higher this conversion rate happens. As such, the more overweight a man is the lower his testosterone levels are and the higher his estrogen. Since testosterone is fat-soluble, it gets sequestered in the fat cells of overweight men and isn't available in the bloodstream to be used.

Support with supplements

- Multivitamin: Be sure you're taking a multi-vitamin formulated for men and preferably food-based, not synthetic, with substantial amounts of vitamins A, E, C, and B6 that play important roles in converting prohormones (precursors) into testosterone.

- Zinc: Crucial for maintaining healthy testosterone levels, zinc is absent in nearly all processed foods. Research shows zinc deficiency and low testosterone go hand-in-hand.[43] When men with low testosterone are given zinc, their levels and sperm count naturally increase.[44] While men with healthy testosterone levels won't get a boost, zinc plays a protective role in keeping levels from falling even after long periods of intense training.[45]

- Vitamin D: Functioning as a steroid hormone in the body, vitamin D, like zinc, is tied to testosterone levels. It has been shown not only to increase testosterone but improve sperm quality as well.[46] When men took 3,300 IU of vitamin D every day, their testosterone levels increased by 20%.[47] Be sure to get some the natural way by being in the sun for about 20 minutes a day.

- D-aspartic acid: A natural amino acid, D-aspartic acid can significantly boost testosterone but only if levels are low. It does this by increasing follicle stimulating hormone and luteinizing hormone which triggers the Leydig cells in the testicles to produce more testosterone.[48] One study found that men with low sperm counts taking D-aspartic acid doubled their levels from 8.2 million sperm per mL to 16.5 million.[49]

- Tribulus Terrestris: Studies have shown men taking this ancient herb experienced improvement with erectile dysfunction and a 16% increase in testosterone.[50] In men with healthy testosterone levels it appears to have no effect.[51]

- Fenugreek: Research found that college men who performed resistance training four times per week experienced higher increases in both total and free testosterone as well as greater fat loss when taking 500 mg per day of the herb fenugreek when compared to men who did not take the supplement.[52] Other research with healthy men between 25 and 52 taking 600 mg of fenugreek per day found substantial increases in libido, sexual performance, energy levels, and sense of wellbeing.[53]

- Ginger: Animal studies have shown ginger increases testosterone and luteinizing hormone levels[54] while others have reported testosterone levels doubling after ginger consumption is doubled.[55] In human studies, infertile men taking ginger supplements saw testosterone levels increase by 17% and luteinizing hormone levels double with a 16% increase in sperm count.[56]

- DHEA: Dehydroepiandrosterone (DHEA) is a naturally occurring hormone in the body and has been extensively researched in its relationship to testosterone. Studies have shown it to increase testosterone by 20% in both healthy men in their 50s and 60s[57] and those with low testosterone at a dosage of 50 mg twice a day.[58]

- Ashwagandha: This ancient Indian herb is known as an adaptogen because of its ability to reduce stress and anxiety. One study with infertile men taking 5 g per day showed testosterone increases of 10% to 22% with 14% of the men's partners actually getting pregnant.[59] Other research has shown that taken with a workout routine ashwagandha increases strength and fat loss and provides a "significant" boost in testosterone from 18 ng/dl to 92 ng/dl.[60]

- Curcumin: As a polyphenol, curcumin is what gives the cooking herb we know as turmeric its yellow color. It helps support testosterone production in several key ways including blocking estrogen at the cellular level,[61] increasing cholesterol processing in the liver,[62] activating vitamin D receptors,[63] accelerating fat loss,[64] protecting testicular cell function from inflammation,[65] and increasing insulin sensitivity.[66] A good maintenance dose is between 500 mg and 1,000 mg per day. Curcumin can be difficult for the body to absorb but research has shown that taking it with a bit of black pepper, perhaps in a smoothie, can increase absorption by up to 2,000%.[67]

- Taurine: Another amino acid taurine is the most abundant free amino acid in the testicles and breast milk. It's also half of all amino acids in heart tissue. Animal studies have shown taurine to protect testosterone from oxidative damage while improving blood flow to the testicles and increasing serum testosterone up to 180%.[68] Other studies show taurine "significantly" raises testosterone, as well as luteinizing hormone (LH) and follicle stimulating hormone (FSH). It's believed this dramatic rise is due to taurine's ability to stimulate human chorionic gonadotropin.[69] Some experts have suggested 5 g three times per day but always check with your doctor before using any supplements.

Testosterone Replacement Therapy

Testosterone replacement therapy (TRT) always remains an option but it should only be considered by men who either have low testosterone from an existing health problem or are at least 55. Finding proper testosterone levels later if life without having a baseline taken 20 or 30 years earlier can be tricky, so expect that there will be changes in dosages along the way based on how you feel.

Be sure to choose bioidentical testosterone over synthetic or conventional options. Bioidentical testosterone is identical in chemical composition to human testosterone and utilized quite easily by the body. Conventional options are synthetic, require a more complex process for their utilization, come with some unnecessary byproducts, and usually end up causing acne and hair loss. Because bioidentical testosterone is identical to your own testosterone, it comes with none of these side effects. It's made from the sex hormone of wild yams and requires only a minor conversion process using heat not chemicals to become identical to human testosterone.

When dealing with hormonal issues, especially sex hormones, I highly recommend finding an endocrinologist of the same sex as yourself. Only a male doctor can truly understand the physical and sexual sensations a male patient describes that he feels in his body. Having this kind of mutual physical life experience to draw from will be absolutely essential for clear communication. Much will already be understood between doctor and patient if they are both of the same sex. This goes for women seeking hormone replacement, as well.

TRT can be administered through creams and gels, time-released skin patches, and subcutaneous pellets. A good doctor will help the patient choose which method works best with his lifestyle. Remember, the idea of TRT isn't to jack your testosterone levels back up to where they were at 25 but to provide just enough to where you're feeling strong, confident, and contented with a good energy level and libido. Think of it as a dusting of testosterone and not a dousing and you'll go in with the right kind of expectations and have excellent results.

Chapter 21

Semen Specifics

It's about more than making babies

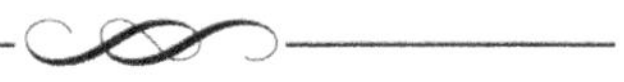

In terms of human physiology, it's easy—and erroneous—to think of each of the body's organs, tissues, and fluids as serving mainly one purpose. The intestines absorb nutrients. The red blood cells carry oxygen. The liver breaks down toxins. While all these statements are true, the fact of the matter is that every part of the body serves many different functions some of which we're only beginning to understand. The human body is integrated to such a high degree that some of the smallest elements carry out or support the most important functions.

One of those elements is semen, the ejaculate produced by men during sexual intercourse. Of particular interest to scientists is the seminal plasma or everything contained in the ejaculate except the sperm cells. Research is showing that semen is a highly complex mixture of ingredients, including female hormones designed for many different purposes. What are female hormones doing in semen?

It turns out that semen does much more than just fertilize an egg cell. Chemicals in seminal plasma through vaginal absorption greatly benefit a woman's health in many ways by providing antidepressant effects, regulating mood, improving cognition, strengthening attachment bonding, coordinating the menstrual cycle, increasing libido, triggering ovulation, ensuring conception, protecting and maintaining a pregnancy, and more.

Synchronizing Cycles

The unique properties of semen piqued the interest of researchers after studies showed that lesbians living together do not experience menstrual synchrony.[1] This is the phenomenon by which women living together in the same house, dorm, or other arrangement will eventually experience synchronized menstrual cycles that happen on or near the same time each month. Evidence shows that menstrual synchrony occurs through the exchange of subtle pheromone cues between the women.[2] This puzzled scientists because it would seem that lesbians, who are in closer and more intimate contact than heterosexual women, would certainly experience the same phenomenon but they do not. Why the difference?

The answer lies in the fact that lesbians have semen-free sex. Scientists now strongly believe based on a large body of research that chemicals in seminal plasma are absorbed through the vagina of sexually active women that trigger pheromones that entrain the menstrual cycles of the other women they live with. In fact, heightened levels of many chemicals in seminal plasma are found in the bloodstream of women in as little as an hour after intercourse.[3]

The process of menstrual synchrony is not only dependent upon a woman being heterosexual but also that she has frequent and unprotected sex, preferably inside a marriage or committed relationship for health reasons. In this context, she will consistently have semen in her reproductive tract that will serve to entrain the cycles of the other women around her. Research underscores this fact by demonstrating that women who live together and are not sexually active or who use condoms, preventing semen from entering their reproductive tract, do not experience menstrual synchrony.[4] With the discovery of semen as the driver behind menstrual synchrony, researchers began wondering if semen exposure affected women's health in other ways and indeed it does.

Antidepressant Effects

One of the most surprising discoveries about semen is its ability to alleviate depression in women. One study asked female college students to rate any depression they experienced based on the Beck Depression Inventory scoring system. Results showed the female students who were not using condoms had the most sex and were significantly less depressed than those who did use condoms. Interestingly, the depression scores for the women using condoms did not differ from those of women who weren't having sex. It's important to note that both the condom and abstinent groups that were more depressed more often had no internal exposure to semen. Further supporting the semen/antidepressant connection was the finding that the more time that elapsed between sexual encounters for the women not using condoms, the more depressed they became. It should be noted that variables such as being in a relationship or single, the length of a relationship, or using oral contraceptives had no impact on the scores.[5]

Researchers believe regular exposure to semen has this effect on women because it contains a host of biological compounds, some at high levels, long known to act as antidepressants and mood elevators. These include prolactin, oxytocin, estrone, estradiol, transcortin, thyrotropin-releasing hormone, serotonin, tyrosine, opioids and 3, 4, dihydroxyphenylalanine, a precursor to dopamine.

In addition to its antidepressant effects, evidence also shows that semen contains properties that affect menstrual regulation, length, and variability, induce ovulation, protect the fertilized egg, maintain a pregnancy, improve cognition, strengthen pair bonding, increase female libido and initiated sexual activity, and alleviate depression or stabilize mood changes related to postpartum, menopause or premenstrual syndrome (PMS). With this in mind, it's worth taking a closer look at these seminal compounds that have such a profound effect on women's health above and beyond reproduction.

Cholesterol & Cortisol

Because cholesterol is the precursor to all steroid hormones, those produced in the adrenal and sex glands, it's no surprise that it's found in semen.[6] Cortisol, the stress hormone formed from cholesterol, also exists in semen at levels about 60% of that found in the blood.[7] Cortisol and its accompanying glucocorticoids accentuate the feel-good effects of dopamine and increase approach or attachment behaviors related to parental care or interpersonal affection. Transcortin, also known as corticosteroid-binding globulin, serves these same purposes and also increases the release of oxytocin, the "love" hormone that creates intense bonding, corticotropin-releasing hormone, and opioids.[8]

Testosterone

Testosterone concentrations in semen are relatively high compared to other compounds.[9] Studies show that the higher seminal testosterone concentrations are associated with better sperm motility. In fact, seminal testosterone concentrations have been found to be significantly higher in men with sperm in their ejaculate than vasectomized men.[10]

About 63% of seminal testosterone and its accompanying androgens are absorbed through the vagina.[11] It is testosterone, not estrogen, that is responsible for the sex drive in women, and it's thought that this absorption contributes to increased libido and female-initiated sexual activity. In fact, research shows that testosterone levels in married women correlate significantly with frequency of sexual intercourse.[12] Other studies support those findings by showing women who do not use condoms have intercourse more often.[13]

Estrogen

Semen contains two types of estrogen, estrone and estradiol, with the level of estrone being about twice that of estradiol.[14] Concentrations of estradiol in seminal plasma are significantly higher than in blood plasma in men.[15] Studies show that estrone administered through the vagina is absorbed rapidly and increases a woman's blood estrogen level by 24 times or 2,400%. Levels remain this high for two hours after exposure.[16] Estradiol administered vaginally has the same dramatic effect with blood levels in women increasing 110 times or 11,000%, also lasting for two hours.[17]

Estrogen along with luteinizing hormone (LH) and follicle-stimulating hormone (FSH) work together to trigger ovulation in women, so it's no surprise that all three of these are contained in semen or that a woman's estrogen levels rapidly increase after insemination. Peak fertility in women coincides with their estrogen peak.[18] Taken together, this means that the effect of semen isn't just to fertilize an egg, but to *actually trigger ovulation* and induce pregnancy.

Researchers hypothesize that the composition of semen evolved to trigger ovulation as a way to increase the odds of impregnation in order to compensate for the fact that humans are no longer cyclical breeders. Every living creature on earth except humans has a definite breeding cycle that is governed by seasons or signals. Many creatures breed in late winter so they can birth their young in the spring and have the summer to raise them. Other creatures like female chimpanzees give very specific signs such as swelling and color changes in their genitalia to signal their ovulation.

Human females give no outward signs of ovulation and have sex year-round. This makes it very difficult for men to synchronize insemination with ovulation in order to achieve impregnation enough of the time to carry on the human species. This is precisely why semen has evolved to trigger ovulation so insemination and ovulation can happen at the same time and increase the odds of pregnancy.

If semen really has evolved to compensate for the lack of cyclical breeding in humans, then it would stand to reason that levels of LH and FSH should be much lower in cyclical breeding creatures because their reproductive success comes from external signs. Research shows this is exactly the case. Not only were levels of LH much lower in chimpanzee semen, but FSH was completely absent.[19]

Estrogen deficits are strongly associated with depression in women, and many studies have shown estrogen therapy improves depression and mood in normal women[20] who have not been diagnosed with clinical or severe depression.[21] It's the presence of estrogen in semen and the dramatic increases it causes in the female bloodstream after exposure that explains why women who have unprotected sex more often experience significantly less depression as we've already seen.

Not only that but estrogen has been effective in treatment of depression related to menopause.[22] In addition, increased unprotected sexual activity has been shown to decrease hot flashes and other menopause symptoms.[23] Research shows 95% of women experience depression or mood disturbances in the days preceding menstruation.[24] Since most women refrain from sex during menstruation it has been suggested that these mood fluctuations may be caused by semen withdrawal. This has been supported by evidence showing an increase in female-initiated sexual activity before and after menstruation.[25]

Although most couples refrain from sex in the weeks after a child is born, sex hormone deficiency or imbalance has been suggested as the cause of postpartum depression. While semen hasn't been studied in this context, postpartum estrogen therapy has been shown to improve severe depression in women.[26] Therefore, sex sooner after birth may provide some relief.

Luteinizing Hormone

Concentrations of LH are extremely high in semen with levels much higher than any other hormone[27] and five times the level found in the blood.[28] In fact, all peptide hormones in semen are either at or below blood levels except LH.

Reasons for the exceedingly high levels of LH in semen are obvious. Not only is LH linked to higher numbers and greater motility of sperm, increasing a man's fertility and chances for conception,[29] but together with FSH works to produce and release eggs in women as both hormones peak at ovulation.[30] Vaginal absorption of these seminal hormones into the bloodstream could act to facilitate or even induce ovulation to maximize the odds of impregnation.

Prolactin

The hormone prolactin has many effects during pregnancy and lactation. Absorption and subsequent increases in a woman's estrogen levels trigger an increase in her prolactin levels, as well.[31] Prolactin has been shown to influence numerous brain functions, including maternal behavior, feeding and appetite, oxytocin secretion, and corticotropin secretion in response to stress.[32] Taken together, it seems prolactin in semen helps entrain the female brain into a maternal mindset in preparation for motherhood. Deficiencies in prolactin have been linked to depression, [33] postpartum depression,[34] and PMS.[35]

Prostaglandins

There are 13 prostaglandins in semen that are rapidly absorbed through the vagina. [36] These compounds assist in ovulation therefore, their presence in semen is thought to serve the same purpose.

In addition, prostaglandins have immunosuppressive capabilities, and it is well-known that a woman's immune function drops slightly during pregnancy so her body does not attack the fetus as an invading entity. [37] A host of cytokines that also have immunosuppressive effects seem to work with prostaglandins to suppress an immune reaction against the sperm cells, giving them time to reach the egg and fertilize it thus further increasing the chances of impregnation. [38] Of course, this means after each encounter of unprotected sex a woman would experience a short period of slightly reduced immunity.

Opioids

Semen contains large amounts of opioid peptides such as β-endorphin that are thought to play a role in immunosuppression.[39] β-endorphin along with calcitonin supports sperm motility with the latter showing a significant correlation.[40]

Enkephalins, another kind of opioid, are found in semen. Along with endorphins they have numerous effects that include decreasing anxiety, elevating mood, analgesia (reducing pain), inducing drowsiness, and immune functions.[41]

Oxytocin

Not only does semen contain compounds that induce the secretion of oxytocin, the hormone that generates feelings of intense bonding, it also contains oxytocin. In addition to strengthening the bond between partners as well as mother and child during birth and lactation, oxytocin increases production of other hormones such as testosterone and prostaglandins. It also influences ovulation and development of the fertilized egg through the blastocyst phase. Oxytocin is also linked to penile erection and female orgasm.[42]

Vasopressin

A peptide hormone, vasopressin is known for its ability to generate defensive feelings and behaviors. These include enhanced arousal, heightened attention or vigilance, and increased aggression.[43] In addition to contributing to sexual attraction between partners, it is thought to also induce behaviors such as protection of a mate and offspring, aggression toward strangers, and defense of home or territory, all the behavioral features we associate with monogamy and parenting.[44]

Proteins

A variety of proteins found in the placenta are also found in semen. These include human chorianic gonadotropin (hCG),[45] human placental lactogen, pregnancy-specific β1-glycoprotein, placental protein 5,[46] and ferritin, a blood protein that contains iron.[47] In many cases, the concentrations of these proteins in seminal plasma are much higher than those found in the blood of men and non-pregnant women and sometimes exceed even the levels of pregnant women.[48] Because these proteins are specifically related to the development and health of the placenta in addition to ferritin providing supplemental iron, which is crucial for women but not men, it's clear that they are working to increase the probability of conception and to help maintain the subsequent pregnancy.

Relaxin

The polypeptide relaxin is produced in the female body during pregnancy by a temporary endocrine structure in the ovaries. In men, it's produced in the prostate and present in semen.[49] Relaxin is also significantly elevated in women nine to 10 days following ovulation.[50] It is thought to play important roles in sperm motility, fertilization, growth of the uterus, preventing preterm labor, cervical ripening, and the facilitation of labor.[51]

The presence of relaxin in semen suggests it also works to manipulate the female reproductive cycle and/or facilitate pregnancy. Because semen contains so many compounds that help induce or maintain pregnancy, it has been suggested that repeated intercourse after conception may help increase positive pregnancy outcomes.[52]

Thyrotropin-releasing Hormone

Produced in the prostate, thyrotropin-releasing hormone is found in high levels in semen.[53] It has been utilized in the treatment of depression[54] and even shown success in treating PMS.[55] Yet another antidepressant compound in semen corroborates why unprotected sex has shown to be beneficial for women's emotional health.

Serotonin

Serotonin's long history of being successful in treating depression is well-documented.[56] Although serotonin does not pass through the blood-brain barrier, researchers estimate that vaginal absorption may allow it to affect peripheral sites, making an indirect impact to alter emotions and behavior. Serotonin also contributes to sperm motility.[57]

Melatonin

The main effect of melatonin is to induce sleepiness or fatigue.[58] It is thought that the inclusion of melatonin in semen is to induce sleep in the female by raising blood levels in order to ensure she remains in a horizontal position for some time after intercourse so as to lengthen sperm retention and maximize the chances for conception. Resuming an upright position too soon after intercourse is known to lessen sperm retention.[59]

Because of its relationship to serotonin, melatonin has also been associated with better moods. Low levels have been associated with people who have attempted suicide and those suffering from Seasonal Affective Disorder.[60] Melatonin deficiency is often seen in bipolar patients.[61]

Neurotransmitters

Neurotransmitters have an enormous impact on human behavior. Norepinephrine and 3, 4, dihydroxyphenylalanine (DOPA) are found in semen at concentrations 19 times and two times higher respectively than in blood levels. [62] A deficiency in neurotransmitters is thought by some to be the underlying cause of depression. Tyrosine is the neurotransmitter that is released in all rewarding behaviors that makes us feel good and reinforces our desire to do or have more of something. When absorbed by the body it is easily metabolized into dopamine. Epinephrine is also present and is involvcd in heightened concentration as well as arousal.[63]

Other Functions of Semen

Regulates / Induces Menstruation

Nearly all previous studies on whether sexual activity affects menstrual regularity did not control for condom use and so made no conclusion about the impact of semen exposure on menstruation, only the sex act itself.[64] Even so, other data has shown a strong correlation between menstrual cycle regularity and intercourse frequency in women who did *not* use condoms but not in those who *did* use condoms. As with depression alleviation, this indicates that the benefit came not from sexual intercourse alone, but the fact that it was unprotected, providing regular semen exposure.

While many compounds in semen can induce ovulation, some have been used to induce menstruation. At first this seems contradictory, but research is showing that semen may well have evolved the ability to change its purpose and even its composition based on the situation in which a male finds his mate.

If a woman in nearing ovulation, hormones in semen can work to trigger an early release of the egg. If she is nearing the end of her cycle, this is far less likely. In this situation, it might be best for the chemical compounds in semen to trigger menstruation in an attempt to terminate the pregnancies initiated by other males. This phenomenon is known as The Bruce Effect and is seen in varying forms in other animal species as part of the reproductive competition to pass one's genes on to the next generation.

Prostaglandins are relatively high during a woman's cycle, and it may be that further elevation from the prostaglandins in semen are enough to trigger menstruation under the right conditions. After all, prostaglandins are commonly used as abortive agents.[65]

Additional research supports this theory. In one study, 25% of men said their partner experienced her period at an unexpected time in her cycle. Of the men, one-third said this occurred just after they began dating or during a visit. Over 25% of women reported a period at an unexpected time with more than one-third saying this occurred after a new sex partner or during a visit. The majority of the women were not using contraceptives and were more likely to report irregular bleeding or inappropriate menstruation when starting a new relationship.

Based on these findings, it is possible that some induced irregular menstruations are actually miscarriages. If this is so, then The Bruce Effect does occur in humans. In the original research, it was found that on beginning a relationship with a new mate, female mice can physiologically abort an existing pregnancy in order to mate with a higher status male.[66]

Enhanced Cognition

Many compounds in semen work to heighten cognition. The presence of epinephrine and norepinephrine support learning and enhanced memory as does vasopressin. Oxytocin increases concentration while estrogen and glucocorticoids also support memory and information consolidation.[67]

At the same time, melatonin contributes to short-term memory.[68] Research shows women who have unprotected sex experience less indecisiveness and have better concentration scores. For those women, concentration difficulty increases in proportion to the length of time between unprotected sexual encounters.[69]

Mutual Health Support

As was stated earlier, the human body is so complex even the smallest element serves many purposes most of which science has yet to discover. The fact that semen serves so many functions beyond fertilization and that they are directly beneficial to the health of women speaks to the symbiotic beauty of human biology and the miraculous relationship between men and women. Consistent and unprotected sexual intercourse as naturally intended within a committed relationship not only creates and supports the health of a pregnancy that will ultimately bring a beautiful baby into the world, but it continues to support the health of both partners for as long as they live together. That indeed is true sexual healing.

Chapter 22

Sex Talk and Timing

How and when to discuss sex with children

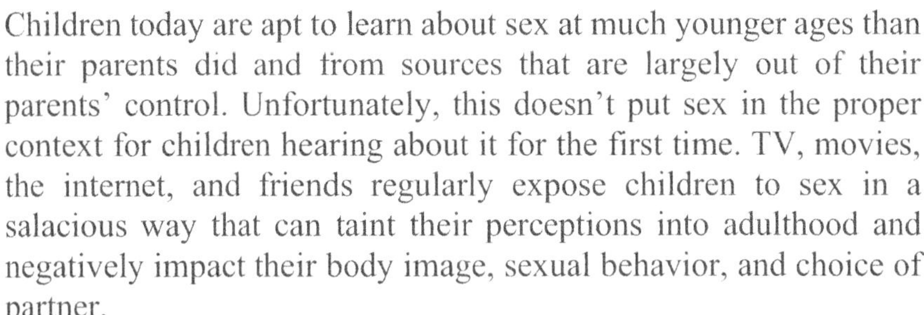

Children today are apt to learn about sex at much younger ages than their parents did and from sources that are largely out of their parents' control. Unfortunately, this doesn't put sex in the proper context for children hearing about it for the first time. TV, movies, the internet, and friends regularly expose children to sex in a salacious way that can taint their perceptions into adulthood and negatively impact their body image, sexual behavior, and choice of partner.

All things considered, including health and sex education classes at school, the best place for children to learn about sex is at home from their parents who care about them the most and understand their individual sensitivities and needs. Even so, most parents think their children don't want to hear from them about sex, but it's actually the opposite that's true.

The Parent Power Survey conducted by Power to Decide found 52% of children between 12 and 15 said their parents had the most influence on them when it came to sex. In contrast, when parents were asked, 60% thought their children's friends held more influence in sexual matters than they did. In reality, only 17% of children said they valued their friends' opinions about sex above their parents. While 28% of teens between 16 and 19 said they valued their friends' ideas on sex more, a slight majority of 32% still said their parents had a bigger influence on them.[1]

Other research found 86% of teens said they talked to both parents and other family members about sex. Most teens reported talking to their mother (95%) followed by their father (38%) and older sister (33%). Aunts, uncles, and a female cousin were mentioned 29% of the time. Responses showed the teens sought out advice for specific reasons that included learning from the adult's life experience, a close relationship with the adult, a feeling that the adult understood the teen, and perceiving the adult as honest and trustworthy.[2]

Talking Points

Anyone can teach the biological facts of reproduction but only parents are in a position to put this information in a context that best suits their children and family's personal, spiritual, or religious values. Although there is no standardized way as to how and when to share information about sex with children, it helps to keep a few things in mind.

1. **Talking to children about sex does not harm their innocence**. Innocence is a function of attitude, not information. A child who understands the dual purpose of sex is to express love and create life maintains a healthy view of it and thus retains his or her innocence. Without this crucial framework, children may be exposed to sex in a way that's abusive or degrading, negatively impacting their view of the opposite sex and themselves.

2. **If you feel overly nervous or inhibited in talking to your child about sex, you might want to review your own attitudes about it.** Perhaps past experience has caused you to feel that sex is bad, dirty, or shameful. It's very important to become conscious of these feelings before they're unconsciously passed on to your children. Recognize this is an issue for you that may require discussion with a therapist to begin your healing process.

3. **Don't wait to share everything you know about sex with your child in a single talk.** Doing so risks waiting until your child has already been influenced by others or overwhelming them with too much information. Facts about sex should be

shared gradually with your child over several years with increasing detail as it becomes age appropriate. The same issue applies with sharing any information with your child as he or she grows, whether it be about handling money, relationships, spiritual values, or anything else. "The talk" is really a series of talks that should begin at a fairly young age.

4. **Give information on a need-to-know basis**. If your five-year-old wants to know how Aunt Susan's baby is going to get out of her belly, she doesn't need to know how it got there. You don't need to provide that much detail at that time. However, if you haven't had any conversations about sex with your eight-year-old, then it's definitely time for you to start the conversation.

5. **Always admit what you don't know**. If you can't answer a child's question, admit that you don't have that information but will look into it and get back with him. Children will respect your honesty and candor more than bluffing and finding out later that you misled them.

Ages 2-3: The right words for genitals such as *penis* and *vagina*.

Ages 3-4: The general place a baby comes from. "Mommy has a uterus insider her tummy. That's where you lived until you were big enough to be born."

Ages 4-5: How a baby is born. "When you were ready to be born, the uterus pushed you out through mommy's vagina."

Ages 5-6: A basic idea of how babies are made. "Mommy and Daddy made you." If the child needs more detail, "A tiny cell inside Daddy called a sperm joined with a tiny cell inside Mommy called an egg."

Ages 6-7: A simple understanding of intercourse. "God/Nature created the male and female bodies to fit together like puzzle pieces. When the penis and vagina fit together, a sperm cell from Daddy swims up to meet the egg cell inside Mommy and make the baby." You can also add, "This is one of the ways mommies and daddies show love for each other."

Ages 8-9: Sex is important and should be experienced in the right context. By this age, children can handle more direct and/or abstract conversations about sex. "Remember when we talked about sex being part of a loving relationship? When someone is forced to have sex when they don't want to, it's called rape, and that's wrong."

Ages 9-11: Talk about the changes that happen with puberty. Also be prepared to discuss sexual topics your child sees in the news as well as things like nocturnal emissions, masturbation, and menstruation.

Ages 12+ Children are starting to form their own ideas about sex. Check in every so often to put the information they're getting into the right context. Be careful not to come off as intrusive. As children get older, you'll want to shift the conversation to focus more on what they're feeling inside that usually drives what they're doing on the outside. Keep children aware of the fact that the sexual images they see in the media aren't real, particularly with regard to how young women are presented, so as to foster a positive relationship between young girls and their bodies.

Avoiding Early Errors

Long before children are aware of what sex is, they love to explore their bodies. Never shame a child who is touching his or her genitals. Even if they cannot talk yet, they will receive the negative energy of your shaming tone and relate it to their sex organs and later their sexuality. Children explore their genitals largely out of curiosity and a need for comfort. Children do, however, have a tendency to touch themselves in public and at other inappropriate times. All that needs to be said is, "This isn't the proper time or place. That's something we do at home in private."

Internet statistics show that 70% of children between seven and 18 have stumbled onto pornography online.[3] If you catch your child on a pornographic site or find out he or she has visited one, try not to get angry. Counteract what has been seen by putting sex back in the proper context and stressing that such sites are for adults. Explain that while you don't approve of pornography, you're not judging your child for viewing it. Always keep family security settings in place on your children's and home internet devices.

At various ages, books can be a great tool to support what you've shared with your child along the way. Be sure to research some and ask friends for recommendations so that you'll have them ready when your children begin asking certain questions. When you pre-plan and start early enough, you can put sex into the proper context for your children in a way that not only preserves its beauty and sacredness but helps them to continue to confide in you as they grow. Knowing they've grown up anchored in your values, you can have peace that they'll make the right decisions in difficult situations and confidence that they'll come to you when they still need guidance.

Chapter 23

X-Rated Exposure

Protecting children from online pornography

The internet revolutionized the world in many ways and some of them not for the better. It used to be that in order to obtain pornography it had to be purchased at an adult store, or ID had to be provided to view X-rated videos from certain rental chains. Even at convenience stores, adult magazines were kept behind the counter and out of public view. Back then, there was a wall between pornography and the public that protected those who weren't interested from unwanted exposure.

Today, that wall has entirely disappeared with the internet providing 24-hour access to every kind of pornography and no one is more at risk of direct or indirect exposure than children. Viewing images they can't possibly understand where dangerous behaviors are detached from any sense of relationship, responsibility, or intimacy affects children in ways that not only rob them of their innocence but affect them well into adulthood.

Pathways to Porn

There are many pathways through which children can inadvertently be exposed to online pornography. A misdirected internet search for a simple word like toy, a misspelled web address, a link or photo from a friend, or even email spam can result in children ending up at websites they never intended.[1] The numbers on how many children are being exposed vary widely. Perhaps this is because some children are either afraid or embarrassed to admit they've seen it. One study found that 42% of adolescents between

10 and 17 reported being exposed either willingly or unwillingly to internet pornography[2] while another study found the rate to be double that at 84%.[3] The good news is that both studies showed that for two-thirds of the children the exposure was unwanted.[4]

Interestingly, when adults are interviewed about their childhood exposure to pornography far removed from the fear of getting in trouble with parents, the numbers are even higher. A study of college students found that 93% of males and 62% of females admitted to seeing internet pornography during adolescence.[5] Another study of college males found exposure for 49% happened before age 13.[6]

External Influences

Although there are many consequences connected to viewing pornography as a young person, few people talk about the developmental risks that come into play, particularly with regard to how a child's personality naturally evolves. My children attended a school based on the Waldorf education system created by Rudolf Steiner. Part of the Waldorf philosophy is to allow a child's imagination and personality to evolve naturally through curiosity and exploration instead of having him or her adopt ideas about the world and who they should be through external images or other people's expectations.

Stories are often told without pictures so children can use their imagination to create their own ideas about things. For the same reason, Waldorf students are not exposed to media until middle school because it's during those crucial early years that they're creating the internal image of who they are. This self-image acts as the foundation for the adults they will become and how they will relate to the world and others around them.

Humans are imitators by nature. When we see something that interests us, we want to have it, participate in it, or learn to do it ourselves. We learn to walk and talk by watching and listening to adults. Likewise, lots of media causes children to imitate the characteristics of the people they see on the screen like Batman or Spiderman instead of using their curiosity and imagination to help their own personality naturally emerge. Avoiding imitation is how children let the superhero already inside them flourish.

This is an important distinction in child development because in this case children aren't looking outside themselves to validate who they are but exploring internally to discover their own gifts and how they can uniquely contribute to the world through them. There is no external stimulus driving them to want to be like anyone else or allowing anyone else to define who they are.

Perverting Perceptions

Like other media, pornography has the same effect of hijacking personality development and imposing foreign norms on us but with regard to sex and our participation in it. The performers in pornographic films aren't portraying an act of love, compassion, or intimacy but almost entirely one of external pleasure. Because the visuals are so intense and hyper-realistic, negative perceptions about sex get quickly embedded in the consciousness of the viewer with regard to how sex is supposed to be, how our bodies are supposed to look, and how we're supposed to behave in an intimate situation. The message is *that's how sex is done.*

This is of particular concern with children because research shows that viewing pornography activates the same regions of the brain related to drug addiction and that the younger the viewer, the greater the neural response.[7] Because of this, children are extremely impressionable when it comes to pornography shaping their perceptions about sex and sexuality.

This imprinting happens through a process researchers call sexual script theory.[8] As children's ideals and expectations get dictated about how sex is carried out in the real world, they begin to see the behaviors, many of which are dangerous or degrading, as normative or acceptable.[9] In fact, research has found a link between watching unprotected sex on screen and going on to have unprotected sex in real life.[10] This supports a survey from the UK that found 44% of boys 11 to 16 viewed online pornography to get ideas about the kinds of sex they wanted to try.[11]

Intentional use of pornography by adolescents and teens puts them at great risk for early sexual activity.[12] Research has shown that the earlier they begin having sex the more prone they are to delinquent behavior, substance abuse, a higher number of sex partners, risky behaviors like group or anal sex, using substances during sex,[13] unprotected sex,[14] higher rates of STDs,[15] and accidental pregnancy.[16]

Currently, the average age for sexual initiation in the U.S. is 17.2 for girls and 16.8 for boys.[17] Since this is the average age, we have to realize that half of the children are having their first sexual experience younger than this, and research shows that most children have experiences with pornography before their first physical encounter.[18] Having sex might make them feel grown up but unfortunately for these children, a large body of evidence consistently shows a negative life trajectory related to early sexual initiation—the younger the age of early intercourse, the more negative the outcomes are in adulthood.[19] Sexting, sending sexual images or messages via text, is very often a gateway into early sexual activity and "significantly associated" with viewing internet pornography, especially for boys.[20]

Sexual Short Circuit

Allowing pornographic images to influence our behavior blocks the natural development of the sexual side of our personality. We lose the ability to express ourselves in a sexual way as a natural extension of who we are because we're consciously or unconsciously trying to imitate something or someone we've seen in a video. We miss out on the beauty that comes from the discovery of sex and how we relate to the other person in terms of energetic and spiritual connection. We can't be present enough to allow those things to happen because we're too busy running a movie in our mind.

We also lose the opportunity to get in tune with our bodies by figuring out what does and doesn't feel good because the goal is always the rush to orgasm. Because we're not mentally present, pornography prevents us from really being in our bodies, as well. The end result is a preoccupied mind thinking, "This is how I'm supposed to give pleasure. This is how I'm supposed to feel pleasure. This is what sex is supposed to look like." A paint-by-numbers approach to sex like this only leaves a person feeling terribly insecure and both people unsatisfied.

Depth or Detachment

Sex is a beautiful and sacred journey two people take together, and even though it may not be the first time for either person, each interaction is an opportunity to make a new discovery and deepen the relationship. This can't happen unless we're focused on our partner and free of performance anxiety and body issues which always come into play because pornography forces us to compare our bodies to those we see in adult films.

Much of this anxiety can be eliminated if we're having sex at the right time and for the right reason, especially if it's the first time. One way to identify the right person, time, and reason to have sex is when you love someone so much you can't express your feelings in words anymore. When you're that in love with someone the little sexual details don't matter right away, and you work the rest out together. In that context, the ability to adapt and change in order to give pleasure to your partner arises naturally out of your love for that person and being present enough to sense their subtle reactions, not a mental checklist.

Without the heart involved in sex, especially for the first encounter, young people run a very high risk of becoming desensitized and incapable of that kind of intimacy because they've been introduced to sex as just a vehicle for physical pleasure. Regular viewing combined with masturbation teaches them that emotions and oftentimes even another person aren't necessary to have their needs met.

A Dutch study of boys 13 to 18 found that the more a boy watched online pornography the more likely he was to have a recreational attitude toward sex and view it as solely a physical function like eating or drinking. In other words, the more they watched pornography the more likely they were to have the "It's just sex" attitude, to see sex as merely a transaction between two people providing a mutual service. The study also found that increased viewing was strongly linked to a belief that it wasn't necessary to have affection for people in order to have sex with them. These attitudes were strongest when the boys perceived the films they were viewing as more realistic.[21] With attitudes like this, children grow up to become part of hookup culture, non-committal pleasure seekers who avoid relationships in favor of casual sex.

This type of dissociated sex robs a person of experiencing true oneness with another human being, which is an important part of understanding our oneness with everything around us, and developing a sense of empathy, vulnerability, and compassion. It also prevents a person from truly connecting with their masculine or feminine energy in a way that only they can express it. Instead, they remain locked in the limitations of physical sensation which soon become monotonous and eventually require increasingly exotic interactions to achieve the same level of pleasure.

Adult Relationship Disaster

Because the adolescent and teenage years are crucial on every level of development, it should come as no surprise that viewing pornography as a young person sets one up for relationship difficulties in adulthood. Not only are pornography and early sexual initiation linked to negative outcomes in adulthood[22] but they're also connected to less life satisfaction overall.[23]

I see so many couples who can't allow themselves to be vulnerable long enough to work out their problems or feelings of isolation so they retreat into pornography, seeking the intimacy and connection they don't have with their partner. Unfortunately, pornography provides no intimacy and their habitual use of it only further prevents real intimacy from happening. Men and women who regularly view pornography eventually develop a stronger preference for pornographic material rather than sexually paired excitement even when their relationship isn't experiencing problems.[24] Pornography drives couples apart. In fact, when a married man begins watching pornography regularly, his chances for divorce double. When married women watch, their chances triple.[25]

Pornography isn't going to help any relationship. What these people need is the courage to be honest and say, "I don't feel seen or heard in this marriage. I don't feel like we're on the same page and moving in the same direction." A conversation needs to be started that no matter how difficult will begin the journey of bringing them back to real intimacy.

Whether it's one or both partners viewing pornography, there is an overwhelming amount of evidence that confirms not only does it decrease sexual satisfaction[26] but it lowers the level of relationship satisfaction, as well.[27] Men who use pornography become less attracted to their spouse.[28] The more pornography they watch the more likely they are to request pornographic sex acts from their partners and conjure pornographic images during sex to maintain arousal.[29] In fact, one study found 20% of men admitted to using porn to stay aroused with their partners and that although pornography increased sexual desire, it lowered sexual satisfaction.[30] This is partly because when men regularly have pleasing sexual experiences with pornography they can begin to need the same kind of stimulation from a partner in order to reach orgasm.[31] This can be a problem if a man's partner is unwilling or unable to perform such acts for whatever reason.

Viewers of pornography often compare themselves to the bodies of the performers they see on screen even though they know (or at least they should) that those bodies are greatly enhanced with breast implants, steroids, and so on. This leads to body image issues and eating disorders for women, especially if they started viewing or became sexually active early.[32] Men are usually less impacted by body issues in society unless they regularly view pornography. In that case, the more a man views pornography the more likely he is to suffer from body image issues regarding muscularity and body fat, as well as performance anxiety in relationships.[33] That's not a surprise considering a study of 15,000 men found the average length of a man's erect penis is 5.2 inches but the typical length for porn stars is more because they are *outliers*, rare exceptions to the rule, and nowhere near the norm.[34] With all this disinterest and insecurity, it's no wonder pornography users increasingly prefer sex alone rather than with their partner.[35]

It's clear that looking at naked men and women other than your spouse engaging in sexual acts leads to breakups, infidelity, and divorce. Regular viewing of pornography beginning at a young age "significantly" predicts relationship instability in adulthood, especially for men.[36] Interestingly, spouses who have an extramarital affair are three times more likely to have used internet pornography.[37]

Preserving Innocence

The best way to protect children against the negative effects of pornography both now and in adulthood is to provide them with a proper set of values that places sex in a spiritual or loving context outside the physical aspects in a way they can understand. The talk should be had at different times throughout adolescence and the teen years so that more detail can be provided as it becomes age appropriate and the message can get reinforced. Activating parental controls on all your child's media devices like cell phone, computer, notebook, and gaming devices is an absolute necessity.

If you find your child has viewed online pornography, don't panic and start yelling. You want your child to trust you and know that he or she can confide in you. Acting from anger and judgment will only leave your child with the impression that sex is bad or wrong. Your goal should be to find out what's going on and if it's a problem. How did the child encounter the pornography? Was it more than once? Does it seem to be a habit? Are there other sites the child has gone to and what has been viewed? Does anyone else at home frequent these sites? Has the child exhibited changes in behavior or mood prior to the incident or been isolating a lot?

It may be that the child has only rarely sought out pornography as a way to satisfy curiosity. In that case, answering any questions the child has, explaining why pornography is harmful for young people, and emphasizing the spiritual side of sex will go a long way toward reframing the issue and redirecting behavior.

Anti-Porn Protocol

Consider these important tips to protect your child from online pornography. Remember that children may still be exposed to pornography by peers whose parents aren't as vigilant, so pay attention to the company your child is keeping. The hyper-sexualization of mainstream media with increasingly explicit images in music videos, fashion advertisements, and so on can also be problematic and may require parental intervention.

- When at home, have your children use the internet in an open area where you can easily see the screen.

- If you have a family computer, create a separate user account for your children.

- Activate parental controls on all search engines and web browsers like Firefox, Google, Chrome, and Safari that filter out websites based on language, nudity, sex, and violence. If you find that's too complicated, you can download and install a search engine designed just for kids to do the same thing like Kiddle or KidSplorer.

- Content filters like Net Nanny and Teensafe provide the same protection but with the added feature of being able to remotely monitor and alter what your child is seeing online in real time. This includes viewing access to your child's emails, texts, and Snapchats. Be careful here that you don't end up violating your child's trust.

- Remember to install or activate content filters on all the child's media, including cell phone, personal computer, and notebook.

- Regularly check your child's browsing history. Content filters do a great job, but it's always best to check up on things once in a while.

- All game systems like PlayStation come with built-in web browsers, but filtering software cannot be installed on the gaming unit. Be sure to follow the instructions that come with the system to create a PIN in order to access the internal web browser.

- Get familiar with the video game rating system and the video games your child is playing. Many with adult themes are very lifelike.

- Activate the privacy setting on all your child's social media accounts, including "restricted mode" on YouTube. Have your child add you as a friend on all social media accounts so you can see what's being posted.

- Don't let your children shop online without you.

- Teach children to keep personal identifying information private.

- If you use pornography be sure to store it in a location where your child cannot get access to it.

When we protect young people from pornography, we protect their innocence which is the key to a life of wonder and discovery. One of the most beautiful discoveries they will ever make is the realization of their sexual selves with the right person, at the right time, and in the right way. Guarding this rite of passage should be a priority for all parents because when it comes to sex, there is no such thing as making a second attempt at a first experience.

Chapter 24

Identity Unknown

Are babies born with no sense of their biological sex?

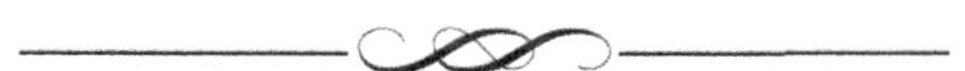

Over the last 20 years or so, the media has made much about the idea of gender identity. Unlike biological sex that determines whether we are male or female based on DNA, gender identity asserts that biological factors are inconsequential and that we can choose our sex from a wide range of intersex categories between male and female based on how we perceive ourselves—even from day to day—because gender identity isn't about biology but "fluidity."

As surprising and unscientific as the gender identity issue may be, it bases its legitimacy on yet another unsubstantiated claim—that children are born with no sense of a specific biological sex and that the roles of male and female are entirely socialized into their minds by stereotypical messaging patterns from parents and society. Babies with XY chromosomes are given trucks and toy soldiers to play with so they're socialized into being boys. Babies with XX chromosomes are given dolls and dresses so they're programmed into seeing themselves as girls. Gender identity advocates claim that without these sex-specific influences children would instead grow up to naturally adopt one of the many gender identities along a "spectrum" as opposed to identifying as strictly male or female.

This is what's known as the Blank Slate Theory; children are born with no personality traits or any sense of themselves and that their psychological development is entirely shaped by the environment around them. Biological factors play no role whatsoever. It's *no* nature and *all* nurture.

Is this true? Do children really have no innate sense of their biological sex? Are environmental factors really that influential? Is there any science at all behind the gender theory? The answers may surprise you.

Identity & Intimidation

It would be easy to dismiss gender identity as an unscientific pop culture fad if it weren't for a very vocal and well-funded minority that has suddenly turned it into a political issue with consequences that are beginning to affect the lives of others whether they subscribe to the idea or not. The New York City Commission on Human Rights passed an ordinance where landlords and employers can be fined $250,000 for failing to address tenants and workers who do not identify as male or female by their "non-binary" pronoun of choice such as ze or hir instead of he or her.[1] Never mind that such utterances aren't even words and have no history or reference in the English language. A slip of the tongue by healthcare workers in California referring to such patients as he or she instead of their preferred pronouns risks a $1,000 fine and one year in jail.[2]

What's going on? The gender identity debate has now turned into a campaign of intimidation and possible violations of freedom of speech against "deniers" who dare to question a theory that has no scientific foundation to support it. It's typical today for the media to negatively brand opposing views so they can be turned into the newest "—isms" and their proponents vilified and ridiculed. Given this trend, it's not surprising that neuroscientists who stand on years of research that show clear differences in the male and female brains are now called "neurosexists." Clever and catchy. This is in spite of the fact that with its January/February 2017 issue, the *Journal of Neuroscience Research* became the first neuroscience journal to ever dedicate its entire issue, 70 articles in all, to the topic of sex differences between the male and female brains with special emphasis on contrasts related to size, connectivity, genetics, epigenetics, cellular and synaptic systems, and more.[3] The editors noted, "The work published in this issue powerfully illustrates that sex matters and that researchers can no longer rely on extrapolation from [male only] clinical studies."[4]

This groundbreaking journal issue was published in response to a policy adopted by the National Institutes of Health (NIH) called Sex as a Biological Variable that officially recognized the fundamental biological differences between men and women and required all its grantees to incorporate an understanding of females into their research. [5] This was an important change for medical research because for centuries it was erroneously assumed that the human body was largely unisex and that it was only the hormones that made humans either inherently male or female. Even when the discovery of DNA changed all of that research was still done almost exclusively on male subjects with the false assumption that the results would also prove to be true in females. We now know from things like how heart attacks present very differently in females (the "silent" heart attack) that women's bodies are profoundly different from men in many ways, especially when it comes to the brain.[6]

Telling Toy Choices

Aside from all the politics, are the male and female brains really different from birth, and do children have an innate sense of their biological sex? The science overwhelmingly says yes.

One of the most thoroughly studied areas of human behavior in sex differences has been with children and toy preference. Decades of research show that children as young as nine months consistently choose sex-specific toys long before they're even aware sex differences exist.[7] To a significant degree, boys choose wheeled toys like race cars, dump trucks, and bulldozers. Girls show a more universal attraction to toys[8] with a clear preference for dolls, plush figures, Lego blocks, or socializing with each other.[9] Meta-analyses of these many studies have confirmed that, "…sexually dimorphic toy preferences reflect basic neurobiological differences between males and females and are not caused solely by socialization, as has been suggested by cognitive-social theories of gender role behavior."[10]

Studies with young rhesus monkeys and toy preference mirror those of human children. Young male monkeys overwhelmingly choose wheeled toys or rough and tumble play, like boys, while young female monkeys, like girls, show more versatility in their toy preference but virtually never choose cars or trucks. These primate studies are significant because young monkeys are not exposed to any alleged sex role stereotyping and yet consistently choose sex-specific toys, proving that the toy choice is biologically based and not socially coerced in both primates and humans. The researchers strongly concluded, "The similarities to human findings demonstrate that such preferences can develop without explicit gendered socialization."[11]

The Binary Brain

Further disproving the assertion that children are born with a unisex, blank slate brain was a groundbreaking study on fetal brain development published in *Developmental Cognitive Neuroscience*. Researchers used functional magnetic resonance imaging (fMRI) and enrichment analyses to examine the growth process of neural networks or functional connectivity (FC) in the brains of 118 fetuses between 25 and 39 weeks of gestation.

The results were astonishing, particularly to those who believe the terms *male* and *female* are meaningless categories based on social constructs. The female fetuses' brains were developing denser neural network connectivity between the posterior cingulate-temporal pole and fronto-cerebellar regions while the male fetuses' brains showed much stronger networks in the intra-cerebellar region. In other words, the male and female brains are literally wired differently and that's why we think differently and have different preferences. The researchers stated, "These observations confirm that sexual dimorphism in functional brain systems emerges during human gestation." They went on to say that these sex-based differences in neural networks form the foundation of our choices and behaviors as children and adults.

> ...fetal brain FC varies with sex. The differential development of FC over gestation in male and female fetuses likely acts as a precursor to sex-related brain connectivity differences observed across the lifespan. Further, the fetal brain networks observed in the present study likely serve as

> the building blocks for nascent neonatal, toddler, and adult networks.[12]

The pattern for traditional sex roles, either male or female, is woven into our brains with different neural networks as we grow in the womb. Of course, this study turns the Blank Slate Theory on its head because it provides physical evidence of sex-based neurological differences in the brains of boys and girls *before birth* and thus free of any influence from society or parents.

Two additional studies provide more weight to the immense body of evidence that continues to show the brains of men and women are distinctly different. A meta-analysis of 126 studies showed men have larger brains with more volume than women.[13] Men have greater neural networks running from front-to-back, while women have greater networks running between hemispheres.[14] This is why men are better at determining direction, perception, hand-eye coordination, and focusing on a single task while women are better with social cognition, communication, and multi-tasking. In fact, the brains of men and women are so different in physical and neurological characteristics that the biological sex of a human brain can be determined with greater than 93% accuracy.[15]

Problematic Parenting

It's difficult to call the Blank Slate Theory junk science because there was never any attempt to pretend it was scientific from the start. Even so, there are those who still cling to it, practicing "gender-neutral" parenting with choices like not revealing their baby's biological sex to anyone after birth so it's not "treated" like a boy or girl, painting the child's room and dressing it in various shades of beige, and giving it abstract toys.

Unfortunately for those parents, Debra Soh, a sexual neuroscientist at York University in Toronto, called such attempts "futile." In an op-ed piece for the *Los Angeles Times* titled, "The Futility of Gender-neutral Parenting" Soh described the bewilderment of gender-neutral parents when their children naturally gravitated toward sex-specific toy choices even without sex-specific toys. Boys would use their imagination to turn pots and pans into bulldozers and dump trucks while girls would ignore their gender-neutral toys and start playing house with each other.[16]

Soh explained that a child having atypical traits or preferences has far more to do with what happens in the prenatal environment, particularly with regard to hormone levels, than the external environment after birth. For example, girls exposed to high levels of testosterone *in utero* develop a condition known as congenital adrenal hyperplasia (CAH). These girls tend to not conform to typical traits and instead prefer toys more common to boys even in spite of their parents offering rewards to choose typical female ones.[17] Based on this evidence, hormone exposure in the womb has far more influence over sex role expression than exposure to people outside the womb.

Soh summed it up by saying gender-neutral parenting was a waste of time because "...the scientific reality is that it's futile to treat children as blank slates with no predetermined characteristics. Biology matters."

A Play on Words

With the evidence so heavily stacked against the Blank Slate Theory, how could the idea of gender fluidity have even taken hold in the public consciousness? Why do some people believe it? The answer lies in creating confusion between two words that have nothing to do with each other: *sex* and *gender*.

The word *gender* comes from the Latin *genus* meaning kind, type, or sort. In biology, genus is a taxonomic classification used to categorize different species of animals (not sexes) into common groups.

Gender is also used to conjugate verbs and articles in some languages, but it does not refer to biological sex. In a language like Spanish, nouns are considered masculine or feminine. For example, *barco* (ship) is masculine and *bicicleta* (bicycle) is feminine. In linguistics, gender refers only to the masculine or feminine classification of a word so that the proper article may be paired with it. In Spanish, *el* is the masculine singular article for the word *the* while *la* is the feminine singular article for the word *the*. Hence, the ship is *el barco* and the bicycle is *la bicicleta*—two different versions of the word *the* based on the gender of the word to which it's referring. Clearly, a bicycle and a ship have no genitalia or chromosomes. *Gender* in linguistics is a mechanism to assist with the proper conjugation of words and is not associated with the biological sex of humans.

The confusion started in 1955 when John Money, a psychologist at Johns Hopkins University, borrowed the word *gender* from linguistics and brought it into the scientific sphere for the first time to refer to the sexual nature of a person's role in society. One of the earliest proponents of "sexual fluidity", Money's implication in using the word *gender* in a scientific context was that if the masculine and feminine nature of certain words could change then human sexual nature could change just as easily and by extension biological sex, too. He established the Johns Hopkins Gender Identity Clinic in 1965 and was an early advocate for what's known as "sex change" or sex reassignment surgery.

Without evidence of any kind, Money's ideas caught on in certain circles. Feminist leader Gloria Steinem once called research into the differences between biological sexes "anti-American crazy thinking."[18] Unfortunately for Money, what he is most well-known for today actually negates his entire theory.

In 1965, Money was at the height of his influence when a tragic accident during a circumcision on a baby boy in Canada left the child's penis irreparably damaged. Money was consulted and oversaw the case. He recommended sex change surgery and that the boy, David Reimer, be raised as a girl. As the years went on, Money was quick to declare the case a total success and proof that "gender" identity is learned.

Entering puberty at age 10, David realized he wasn't a girl. At 15, he began to live as a boy but suffered from severe depression because of his ordeal for the rest of his life. At 38, he committed suicide. John Money had no comment. Today, Money's work is now highly and rightly criticized.

Confusion Continues

Money died in 2004, but the confusion he wrought between *gender* and *sex* lives on. In fact, it thrives. Nearly everyone in the media and politics sees both words as interchangeable and mostly use *gender* where the word *sex* should be applied.

In fact, research shows for most of written history *gender* was virtually never used to refer to biological sex. In 1988, *sex* was used 10 times more often than *gender* in medical literature and mass media communications when referring to men or women. By 2000, *gender* was being used interchangeably with *sex* to such a degree that it is now used nearly twice as often when the proper word for the context should be *sex*. Incorrectly using *gender* as a synonym for *sex* has become such a problem in the medical industry that many physicians have raised the alarm, fearing how such confusion can affect the reputation, legitimacy, and accuracy of research.[19] Hence, the idea that biological sex is changeable is endlessly and erroneously perpetuated through this unconscious word switch.

The fact that there are only two biological sexes based on DNA and yet there are allegedly dozens of different "genders" should be proof enough that gender and sex are not the same thing. In fact, the gender identity idea is so baseless that no one really knows how many there are. The New York City Commission on Human Rights says there are 31[20] while you can sign up on Facebook under any one of 58 gender identities that include titles like genderfluid androgyne, agender version gendervoid, demiboy, or even "something else entirely." [21] Clearly, that's not scientific terminology. Yet, healthcare workers in California are being threatened with fines and jail time if they don't use these pop culture terms with their patients.

Taking a word that belongs in a linguistic context and placing it in a scientific context makes as little sense as taking terms that define speed in music theory and placing them in a scientific context to refer to speed across space and time. Terms defining speed or tempo in music can't be used in a scientific way to determine speed across space and time because whether a piece of music is played moderately fast (allegretto) or very fast (prestissimo) is entirely dependent on the opinion of what a musician determines those speeds to be. They are relative and immeasurable, and yet the principles of science tell us that for something to be considered a scientific fact it must be observable, measurable, and repeatable.

Therefore, you won't find an allegretto sign along the highway to tell you *exactly* how fast to drive nor is there any biological test that can measure "gender" in human beings.

Much the same thing has happened with the confusion between the words *ethnicity* and *race. Ethnicity* refers only to the non-biological characteristics of a people such as their cuisine, clothing, music, religion, holidays, and language whereas *race* refers strictly to the DNA markers that classify a person as part of a biological racial group such as Caucasian or Asian. For example, a Caucasian man could move to Japan and take on all the ethnic elements of a Japanese lifestyle but it would never make him Asian or Japanese. Even so, nearly everyone in the media uses the word *ethnicity* when they should be saying *race*. One comes from anthropology and the other from biology, once again, two entirely different contexts.

The best way to end this confusion and begin to re-educate people is to use the right word in the right context. Unless you're studying a language like Spanish or Italian that involves word conjugation, there is no reason to use the word *gender* at all. In that case, simply say biological sex or sex when referring to a person as male or female.

Complement Not Compete

The more it's examined the clearer it becomes that the Blank Slate Theory isn't based in biology but political ideology, the misconception that if men and women are ever to be truly "equal" then they have to be the same. This stems from the illogical fear that as neuroscience continues to prove that men and women are not the same then they can never be "equal." Just more confusion of terms. Equality isn't sameness; that's cloning.

Neuroscience continues to show that the male and female brains are the same or similar on average in many respects and yet very different a little to a lot in other respects. We've covered some of these discoveries in other chapters. These findings are incontrovertible and won't be going away in the future but will only continue to grow. Does that mean that men are better than women and women are better than men at certain things? Yes. Does it mean that men or women are better overall? No.

Success in life is about cooperation, and men and women are built to complement each other through their biological strengths not compete with each other or try to be the same which is impossible anyway. Men and women are better together distinctly *as men and women*. It's awe-inspiring to know that this primal partnership is so vital to the human species that our sense of maleness or femaleness is neurologically woven into our brains even before we're born. Let's celebrate it instead of pathologize it.

Chapter 25

A Lie of the Mind

Transgenderism as mental illness

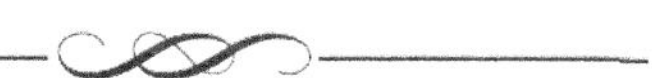

How do we determine who we are? Forming an identity is the foundation of human existence. Once we answer that question for ourselves, we can interact with the world in a way that's congruent with our identity. Our place and function in society become clearer. Life makes sense as we move forward adopting viewpoints and taking actions that continue to strengthen our sense of self.

In forming our identity, no other aspect is more important than biological sex. It's our primal identity and cuts to the very core of who we are. Long before we identify with external things like a religion, political party, job title, or even our race we come to understand as toddlers that there are only two kinds of human beings on earth, males and females, and we are either one or the other. That realization is the foundation and beginning of self-awareness.

When there is confusion between a person's sexual identity and their biological sex as is the case with transgender people, it generates great stress throughout every aspect of their lives. They can't live fully and freely because there is a significant psychological conflict between who they are with regard to their biology and who they believe themselves to be.

The plight of transgender people deserves great compassion but how their struggle is being met by medicine is of great concern. Unfortunately, well-funded special interest groups have made politics the center of the issue and under the guise of civil rights pressured the medical establishment into fast-tracking transgender adults into radical, life-altering surgeries and pubescent children into cross-hormone therapy that they later grievously regret. This is happening all while increasing numbers of transgender people are searching for ways to "de-transition" as mounting evidence continues to show transgenderism is a mental illness in desperate need of psychological treatment, not surgery.[1]

Politics & Semantics

Since the 1970s, transgender people were diagnosed with Gender Identity Disorder (GID) as described in the American Psychiatric Association's (APA) *Diagnostic and Statistical Manual of Mental Disorders* (DSM-5), the official compendium of all known mental illnesses. After heavy lobbying of the APA by special interest groups that claimed transgender people suffered a social stigma from the word *disorder* in their diagnosis, the organization changed the name of the condition from GID to gender dysphoria in 2013.[2]

The change caused much celebration among transgender advocates assuming that transgenderism was no longer a mental illness as if someone could just declare a thing on paper and then make it so. In fact, the name change was little more than medical wordplay. The transgender community didn't want to be labeled "disordered" but removing their condition entirely from the DSM-5 as a mental illness would have made them ineligible for coverage for medical services. With this in mind, the APA played semantics by giving the condition a new name without the offending word while keeping it as a classification in the DSM-5. In other words, just changing the name of the condition changed nothing. As long as transgenderism can be diagnosed under a classification of the DSM-5, the official reference guide for mental disorders, it is considered a mental disorder.

Reality Disconnect

Gender dysphoria refers to the clinically significant stress, anxiety, or depression that arises from personally identifying with one of the two sexes that is opposite a person's biological sex, a man who perceives himself and identifies as a woman or a woman who perceives herself and identifies as a man. In principle, it's very similar to another mental disorder, body dysmorphic disorder

(BDD) where a person is unable to see their body objectively as it is and instead obsesses on some aspect or part that they feel needs fixed or changed. A subgroup of this condition includes muscle dysmorphia when bodybuilders become obsessed with exercise and steroids because no matter how big they get they still see their bodies as small when they look in the mirror. This also applies to anorexia where no matter how much weight one loses, they only see a fat person in the mirror and so the obsession with dieting goes on. Like a transgender man who perceives himself as a woman, there is a fundamental inability to recognize objective reality in all these conditions.

Those who believe that transgenderism is now no longer a mental illness mistakenly liken the GID name change to the removal of homosexuality from the DSM-5 in 1987 as a similar step forward in the march toward sexual rights except that isn't an accurate comparison. Homosexuals do not suffer from an inability to recognize objective reality. When they look in the mirror, there is no conflict with what they see and how they feel with regard to their biological sex. A gay man still sees himself as a man and feels like a man, and lesbians see and feel themselves to be women. In addition, homosexuality was entirely removed from the DSM-5 while transgenderism was simply renamed.

It's the inability to recognize and reconcile with objective reality that's at the heart of transgenderism. The inability to recognize reality involves a self-delusion. Unfortunately, countless governmental, medical, and social institutions not only encourage but enable this condition for their own political and financial gain. In fact, the U.S. Supreme Court recently declared transgenderism to be a protected class under Title VII of the Civil Rights Act of 1964.[3] This marks the first time a mental illness was normalized by judicial edict.

How can this be? It would be obvious to any rational person that an adult male who identified himself as an 8-year-old child, alien from another planet, or even an animal was suffering from some sort of mental illness. On the other hand, when he identifies as a woman nothing is out of order? I make this comparison not to disrespect the struggle of transgender people but to demonstrate the absurdity and danger of normalizing it as research continues to show increasing numbers are committing suicide, especially after their surgeries. This is happening as the medical industry charges over $100,000 for each "transition" and transgender people continue to be unwittingly used as political pawns.[4]

Pre-Existing Mental Illness

A clinical review from the Department of Psychiatry at Case Western Reserve University of the university's Gender Identity Clinic found that 90% of transgender patients "...had at least one other significant form of psychopathology...[including] problems of mood and anxiety regulation and adapting to the world." Some also had "...persistent and significant regrets about their previous transitions." The researchers expressed great concern about the agencies claiming to help transgender adults and how the issue was being manipulated for political and financial gain at the expense of the patients.

> This finding seems to be in marked contrast to the public, forensic, and professional rhetoric of many who care for transgendered adults...Emphasis on civil rights is not a substitute for the recognition and treatment of associated psychopathology. Gender identity specialists, unlike the media, need to be concerned about the majority of patients and not just the ones who are apparently functioning well in transition.[5]

Studies from Sweden and the Netherlands also confirm that as many as 90% of transgender people suffer from mental disorders related to depression and anxiety and that their cross-gender identification is a secondary effect that arises out of "other psychiatric illnesses, notably personality, mood, dissociative, and psychotic disorders." [6] In fact, these serious mental disorders were identified in 79% of all transgender people.[7]

As evidence continues to mount that transgender people overwhelmingly suffer from one or more of these Axis I disorders,[8] researchers are urging the medical establishment to focus on helping patients develop coping skills so they might better adapt to the world and their place in it.[9] Unfortunately, their call to action has fallen mostly on deaf ears as the mental health needs of transgender people go entirely unaddressed and they commit suicide in increasing numbers.

Suicide Epidemic

All the psychopathologies that occur in tandem with cross-gender identification are highly associated with suicide.[10] Because of this, it's an unfortunate fact that as transgender people struggle to adapt to their bodies and their place in the world, they commit suicide at much higher rates than the general public. Unfortunately, these numbers increase exponentially *after* surgery which changes virtually nothing for them on a psychological level.

The longest and most comprehensive follow-up study on post-operative transgender people occurred in Sweden, a culture strongly supportive of transgenderism, and examined all cases of patients who underwent sexual "reassignment" surgery from 1973 to 2003. At some point in their lives 41% of transgender people will attempt suicide compared with 4.6% of the larger population.[11] According to the Swedish study, after surgery, the suicide rate for transgender people is 19 times the rate of the general public with the highest risk in male-to-female patients.

As such, transgender people have a much higher mortality rate than the general public which the researchers attributed mostly to completed suicides. At the same time, transgender people were found to have a death rate from cancer and cardiovascular disease 2.5 times higher than control groups. Although researchers did not speculate, it may be that these increases are due to the long-term effects of cross-hormone use. The study also showed psychiatric hospitalization was triple the rate of non-transgender people.[12]

An important point made in the study was that the majority of these suicides and diseases occurred 10 to 15 years after surgery when physicians are no longer following patients and the initial post-operative euphoria of "becoming" the opposite sex has worn off. Long after the media stories celebrating post-operative transgender people have left the front page their darker and deeper struggle begins but no one is paying attention anymore.

Surgery No Solution

As the political campaign supporting transgenderism rolls on, the medical evidence continues to mount showing that physical treatments like surgery and hormone therapy for what is fundamentally a mental illness make no impact on the long-term quality of life for transgender people. A review of the literature on treatment for gender dysphoria by the APA found, "The quality of evidence pertaining to most aspects of treatment in all subgroups was determined to be low."[13]

An analysis of more than 100 international medical studies of post-operative transgender people found "no robust scientific evidence that gender reassignment surgery is clinically effective." The lead researcher at Birmingham University in Britain found that studies supporting surgery for transgender people were poorly designed with skewed results that were biased toward "changing" sex with no evaluation of other treatments such as long-term counseling or if cross-sex identification lessened over time. Other studies were unsound because they lost track of over half the participants, many probably due to suicide. Because of this, researchers gave the studies supporting transgender surgery the lowest rating for quality.[14] In their final report, they stated:

> Statistically significant improvements have not been consistently demonstrated by multiple studies for most outcomes...Evidence regarding quality of life and function in male-to-female adults was very sparse. Evidence for less comprehensive measures of well-being in adult recipients of cross-sex hormone therapy...was sparse and/or conflicting. The study designs do not permit conclusions of causality and studies generally had weaknesses associated with study execution, as well. There are potentially long-term safety risks associated with hormone therapy but none have been proven or conclusively ruled out.[15]

While Medicare and Medicaid have not issued a National Coverage Determination (NCD) on a blanket approval for transgender surgery, the agencies will still pay for those procedures on a case-by-case basis. Even so, those agencies expressed grave concerns about the success of surgery in a memo stating:

> Overall, the quality and strength of evidence were low due to mostly observational study designs with no comparison groups, subjective endpoints, potential confounding...small sample sizes, lack of validated assessment tools, and considerable loss to follow-up...The majority of studies were non-longitudinal, exploratory type studies...or did not include concurrent controls or testing prior to and after surgery...studies did not demonstrate clinically significant changes or differences in psychometric test results after [gender reassignment surgery].[16]

Of course, the failure of surgery to help transgender peopled isn't a new discovery. In 1979, 13 years after the first transgender surgery was performed in 1965, endocrinologist Charles Ihlenfeld, who had treated more than 500 post-operative transgender patients with cross-hormone therapy, confided in a letter to fellow endocrinologist Harry Benjamin, "There is too much unhappiness among people who have the surgery. Too many of them end as suicides. Eighty percent who want to change their sex shouldn't do it."[17]

Later he would write in *Transgender Subjectivities: A Clinician's Guide*, "Whatever surgery did, it did not fulfill a basic yearning for something that is difficult to define. This goes along with the idea that we are trying to treat superficially something that is much deeper."[18] Dr. Ihlenfeld eventually left endocrinology to pursue a residency in psychiatry.

Bravery & Backlash

Dr. Paul McHugh, former Psychiatrist-in-Chief at Johns Hopkins Hospital and Distinguished Service Professor of Psychiatry, made waves in the media when his op-ed was published in *The Wall Street*

Journal titled Transgender Surgery Isn't the Solution: A drastic physical change doesn't address under-lying psycho-social troubles.[19] In the article, McHugh stated that transgender surgery is never medically necessary or ethically defensible and that surgeons performing such procedures are "cooperating with delusional thinking" likening the practice to giving liposuction to anorexic patients.

After reviewing decades of transgender cases at Johns Hopkins Hospital, Dr. McHugh found patients were no better adjusted to their world after surgery stating, "They had much the same problems with relationships, work, and emotions as before. The hope that they would emerge now from their emotional difficulties to flourish psychologically had not been fulfilled."[20] With this evidence, Dr. McHugh was instrumental in getting transgender surgeries stopped at Johns Hopkins Hospital in 1979.

Even so, after backlash from Dr. McHugh's op-ed and pressure from the Human Rights Campaign and other LGBTQ organizations, transgender surgeries were resumed at Johns Hopkins Hospital in 2016 after 37 years. In a press release, the hospital celebrated the return of what it called "gender-affirming" surgery."[21] The new feel-good title for the surgery only underscored that the hospital knew it was impossible to change or even "reassign" biological sex. The only thing the surgery was affirming was the delusion of its patients.

Targeting Children

Regardless of the softer, emotional labels the healthcare industry and media prefer to give transgender surgery, it doesn't eliminate any of the dire risks that come with it. Dr. McHugh insists, "...policymakers and the media are doing no favors either to the public or the transgendered by treating their confusions as a right in need of defending rather than as a mental disorder that deserves understanding, treatment and prevention." This is particularly important because Dr. McHugh cites two studies from Vanderbilt University and London's Portman Clinic of Children that show up to 80% of young people who express transgender confusion about their biological sex lose those feelings over time.[22]

Taking a similar bold step, the American College of Pediatricians (ACP) issued a scathing indictment against the push for transgender medical interventions for children titled Gender Ideology Harms Children. In it, the ACP cited the APA's own findings published in the DSM-5 that state 98% of boys and 88% of girls experiencing transgender confusion eventually accept their biological sex naturally after passing through puberty.[23] It also cited many studies documenting the dangers and permanent damage done to children from cross-hormone therapy and puberty blockers such as sterility, hypogonadism, stunted growth, cardiac disease, blood clots, diabetes, and cancer. In the end, the ACP stated that, "No one is born with a gender. Everyone is born with a biological sex...Conditioning children into believing a lifetime of chemical and surgical impersonation of the opposite sex is normal and healthful is child abuse."[24]

Compulsory Coverage

Unfortunately, increasing numbers of transgender people of all ages are being pushed into cross-hormone therapy and surgery by political cheerleaders and medical enablers. Medical tracking data have revealed that transgender surgery has tripled in recent years with 48,000 people, half of them under age 30, undergoing the procedure since 2016.[25] This drastic increase is thought to be the result of the Affordable Care Act barring discrimination based on gender identity and in effect mandating coverage of transgender services by nearly all insurance companies.[26]

Sadly, the rush into irreversible medical interventions has ruined the lives of most post-operative transgender people. Once they eventually come to accept their biological sex or realize surgery wasn't the emotional panacea it was promised to be it's too late and the devastation sets in. With the amputation of healthy body parts there is no way back to their former lives or selves in spite of consultations with surgeons in an attempt to "de-transition." Intense regret leaves them with nowhere to turn because expressing second thoughts about transgenderism in any way is often shouted down as intolerant, bigoted, trans-phobic, and infringing upon the sexual health rights of others.

Devastating Regret

Because the political, medical, and media alliance promoting transgenderism is broad, well-funded, and powerful, getting actual statistics on how many post-operative transgender people regret their decision is nearly impossible. Those who do dare to express their regret openly are either humiliated in the press or regularly accused of not *really* being transgender to begin with.

One of those people is Walt Heyer who, in order to escape the pain of early childhood trauma, adopted a female identity that arose out of what he would later learn was dissociative identity disorder. At 42, he had surgery and lived as a woman for eight years after which he realized that it was impossible to truly become a woman. It was that discovery that helped him begin to accept his biological male sex. After intense therapy to deal with surgery regret, he now helps other "regretters" share their stories and provides assistance for them to move forward with lives that have purpose and meaning via his online service sexchangeregret.com.

Because Heyer stepped out of the shadows with his sex change regret, others are slowly gaining the courage to do the same. In his book *Trans Life Survivors*, 30 people share their heartbreaking stories and what it cost them to come out of the trans regret closet.

Urologists such as Miroslav Djordjevic who specialize in transgender surgery have seen an increase in "reversal" surgeries, particularly in trans women who want their male genitalia back. Dr. Djordjevic said these patients display high levels of depression and suicidal thoughts. This isn't surprising since male-to-female transgender people have the highest suicide rates. He told *Newsweek*, "It can be a real disaster to hear these stories."[27]

A Swedish documentary titled *Regretters* gained a lot of attention when it followed two transgender women who returned to living as men in their 60s.[28] As the social conversation about transgenderism slowly expands beyond the accepted narrative, people are feeling more emboldened to share the details others don't want us to hear, as one regretter told *The Guardian*.

> Transsexualism was invented by psychiatrists. You fundamentally can't change sex. The surgery doesn't alter

> you genetically. It's genital mutilation. My 'vagina' was just the bag of my scrotum. It's like a pouch, like a kangaroo. What's scary is you still feel like you have a penis when you're sexually aroused. It's like phantom limb syndrome. It's all been a terrible misadventure. I've never been a woman, just Alan.[29]

For some transgender people, regret happens immediately after surgery. For others, regret develops slower as disillusion sets in over the coming years. This was the case for Los Angeles sportswriter Mike Penner who shocked everyone after announcing in his column that he would be returning from a three-week vacation as "Christine Daniels."[30] After living as a woman for a year and without explanation, he decided to resume living as a man. Sadly, the post-operative struggle was too much for him and he committed suicide.[31] Penner's funeral was private to keep out the media. Some in the LGBTQ community had their own memorial service, but it was only for "Christine Daniels" and not Mike Penner.

In spite of these heartbreaking stories, transgenderism advocates insist that transgender people living in their post-op bodies for decades are well-adjusted and the real success stories. This isn't entirely true, and longevity is no barometer for happiness for a post-op transgender person. Famous tennis player and ophthalmologist Richard Raskind had surgery to become Renee Richards in 1975. After living nearly 25 years as a woman, he shared this with *Tennis Magazine*:

> If there was a drug that I could have taken that would have reduced the pressure, I would have been better off staying the way I was—a totally intact person. I know deep down that I'm a second-class woman. I get a lot of inquiries from would-be transsexuals, but I don't want anyone to hold me out as an example to follow. Today there are better choices, including medication, for dealing with the compulsion to cross dress and the depression that comes from gender confusion. As far as being fulfilled as a woman, I'm not as fulfilled as I dreamed of being. I get a lot of letters from

> people who are considering having this operation…and I discourage them all.[32]

In a later interview with *The New York Times* titled The Lady Regrets, the reporter described Richards this way, "…as she wearies of the interview, her body language seems to become more traditionally male, suggesting an athlete who is wearying of the game."[33]

Although no one is about to fund a large, long-term study of transgender surgery regret for obvious reasons, we can get a credible idea of how serious the problem is just based on existing evidence. When we consider that post-operative transgender people have a suicide rate 19 times higher than the general public and the fact that 65% of people who have standard cosmetic surgery end up regretting it, the level of regret from procedures as drastic as transgender surgery must be very high regardless of what the media says.[34]

Exploring Origins

It was once thought that abnormalities with androgen receptors involved in sexual differentiation as happens with hermaphroditism (a birth defect resulting in the development of both male and female sexual genitalia) might be at the heart of transgenderism. Even so, research of men with transgender feelings has shown no genetic abnormalities whatsoever. Researchers stated, "This gender disorder does not seem to be associated with any molecular mutations of some of the main genes involved in sexual differentiation."[35]

This evidence, along with the fact that the DSM-5 tells us the overwhelming majority of people lose their transgender feelings over time as well as the mounting cases of post-operative regret, underscores the reality that transgenderism is mental in origin, not physical. It therefore demands psychological intervention, not surgery or hormones.

Okay, but how does transgenderism happen? Once again, there is virtually no research in this area. Because the existing medical establishment doesn't see transgenderism as a problem, it doesn't study it in that respect.

In Walt Heyer's case, he believes that escaping the pain of childhood trauma through an alternate identity is one way it happens. A person can't get further away from his or her own identity than adopting that of the opposite sex. He stated:

> Advocates and trans-clients fear that if a psychologist or a psychiatrist looks too deeply into the patient's psyche, they could discover the presence of a disorder that, if properly treated, would take away the dream of sex change, a fantasy they nurtured most of their lives. Living in denial is often a means of escape, a way to avoid looking back at early childhood events and doing the hard work of dealing with a painful past. The causes of these disorders lie buried so deep, and stirring them up leads to such high levels of anxiety, that changing one's identity and appearance—while extreme—seems preferable. Thirty-three years ago, I underwent gender-reassignment surgery only to discover it was a temporary reprieve, not a solution to the underlying comorbid disorders.[36]

More mental health professionals are starting to suspect that the phenomenon can happen subconsciously as a way to escape all sorts of challenges in life. Nancy Verhelst of Belgium was devastated after her transgender surgery transformed her into "Nathan" saying the procedure turned her into "a monster." Years later, she realized her feelings of wanting to be a man had arisen from the rejection of her mother who always preferred her brothers. Physicians eventually put Nancy to death at her request under the country's euthanasia law.[37]

Dr. McHugh believes that in many male-to-female cases the men cannot come to terms with their homosexuality and subconsciously seek becoming a woman as a way to ease the moral conflict between their sexual orientation and their biological sex. He also suspects that cross-dressing along with an obsession to inhabit the female form too deeply may create confusion in some men.[38]

Research from Brown University found that the media was a major force in creating transgender confusion, especially in young people. It went so far as to call transgenderism among the young a fad that young adults attached themselves to because it was hip and driven by "peer contagion."[39] Outrage from transgender advocates caused the university to remove the study from its own site.[40]

Whose Truth?

When politics and profit are put before patients, the most vulnerable people always suffer. This is undoubtedly the case with transgender people. When there is such a clear disconnect between objective reality and personal identity, psychological intervention should be the first and only course of action. Anything else is tantamount to malpractice. Dr. McHugh is correct when he states:

> Sex change is biologically impossible. People who undergo sex-reassignment surgery do not change from men to women or vice versa. Rather, they become feminized men or masculinized women. Claiming that this is a civil-rights matter and encouraging surgical intervention is in reality to collaborate with and promote a mental disorder.[41]

Yet, the healthcare establishment, media, and advocacy groups continue to urge transgender people to "live their truth." Where will that lead them when their truth is based on a lie of the mind?

Epilogue

The courage to lead

We live in interesting times. As the world becomes more politically and socially polarized into an ever-increasing number of interest groups, it seems everyone has something to say. The problem is that except for the members of one's own in-group, no one wants to hear it. In a world where tolerance is supposed to be the order of the day, we're becoming increasingly intolerant of anyone who happens to hold a view that challenges our own. It's so bad that laws are being enacted the world over to limit and even criminalize the free expression of certain thoughts and ideas just because someone else doesn't like them.

It's no longer enough to refuse to hear viewpoints that oppose our own. We must make sure no one else hears them, as well. As such, society now seems compelled to make public examples of heretics who dare to challenge the status quo by either having them arrested, shaming them into silence through merciless ridicule in the press, destroying their career, or any combination of these persecutions. This is cancel culture as we've come to know it in the 21st century, a professional assassination of someone's career and credibility to act as a warning to others; dare to speak out against the mainstream narrative in science, medicine, politics, or anything else and face getting cancelled from modern society, too. In a similar way, ancient civilizations used shunning and making someone an outcast to enforce conformity.

In any case, the freethinker soon comes to understand that expressing thoughts outside narrowly defined socially acceptable parameters will not be tolerated. With enough of a backlash, the offender will eventually stop thinking such thoughts and fall back in line. Except in rare cases of a few courageous people, this kind of pressure works almost every time.

In no profession is the resistance to new ideas and pressure to conform greater than in medicine. There is simply one way of doing things, one philosophy of patient care, and it will not be challenged without great consequences. Any physician who takes their vocation of healing seriously cannot remain silent when the health and wellbeing of patients is at stake. Free speech is crucial to any civilized society and particularly in medicine which hasn't cured or eradicated a single disease in nearly a century.

If we intend to keep our children and grandchildren from suffering from the same chronic diseases that plagued the five or six generations before them, we must allow the free exchange of ideas to flow, especially when it comes to medical research, treatment, and prevention strategies. This means sharing ideas that many might find unacceptable today but that in a generation could easily be viewed as standard care.

How else does discovery happen and the world move forward without humans challenging each other's ideas? As George Orwell author of the dystopian novel *1984* said, "If liberty means anything at all, it means the right to tell people what they don't want to hear."

Many leaders in medicine don't want to hear alternative healthcare theories because they are financially invested in the existing superstructure of corporatized healthcare and thus dependent on its existence for their livelihood. From doctors, nurses, lab technicians, and researchers to university professors, medical center administrators, and journal editors, tens of millions of people rely on the existing system for their personal security and professional reputations. Billions of dollars in research grants, pharmaceutical sales, surgical interventions, and treatments are wholly dependent on doing things the way we've been doing them for nearly 100 years. It's no wonder the medical powers-that-be feel threatened every time something new is suggested that might compete with the existing system and draw away dollars.

While modern medicine has improved greatly with regard to diagnostics over the years, it still holds a dismal record when it comes to actually curing the diseases it has become so much better at diagnosing. That's because the philosophy and approach to medicine haven't changed since there is so much profit to be made from the existing model. Billion-dollar incentives prevent any new ideas from getting past the information gatekeepers even if those ideas mean saving more lives.

I've come to understand through firsthand experience that you can't be a true healer today and not be a nonconformist. As diseases like cancer and neurodegenerative disorders continue to ravage the present generation just as they did in the past, continuing to do things the way they've always been done is not only irresponsible but negligent. It's now incumbent upon physicians as healers to say it's time to find another way. Taking such a stance requires stepping away from the crowd and forging a new path as a trailblazer, a reluctant leader who isn't so much self-declared but chosen by fate and necessity to ignite the next evolution in healthcare.

It's never been any other way. All the greatest scientists, physicians, and philosophers from Galileo onward were threatened, professionally ruined, and even jailed for expressing ideas that we take for granted today. To be a healer means to be a leader whether one likes it or not. To be a leader also means to be alone, at least until your idea gains favor, because society is overwhelmingly populated with followers, people driven by polls not passion, consensus not courage. An old Polish proverb states that eagles fly alone but sheep flock together. This is how I've chosen to run my life and my medical practice, flying alone and showing others a new way regardless of those that would seek to ground me.

I wholly believe in patients taking charge of their health through dietary and other lifestyle choices. This includes everything we choose to put in or on our bodies such as colognes, personal care products, and even clothing. We have far more control over our health than we think we do, and I believe in empowering my patients in this way as much as possible.

Often the cumulative effect of the choices we make every day over time is the cause of the diseases that seem to "just happen" later in life. Over 30 years in medicine has taught me that no disease just appears out of the blue and that there is far more we can do from a preventative standpoint to secure our health later in life if we have the proper information to help us make the right choices early on.

I've made many public statements to this effect in my books, on various websites, and in interviews. I've demonstrated the power of resolving old emotional issues, herbal supplements, detoxification, and countless natural therapies when it comes to awakening the body's own healing process through real-world experiences with my own patients. Unfortunately, these stories of healing that should have been met with excitement too often triggered a backlash from the medical establishment and its guardians in the media.

To say that I've been excoriated in the press at certain times would be putting it mildly. I've been called a kook and a guru who was "sparking outrage" by pushing "debunked" myths that have long been "scientifically discredited." They've painted me as everything from the Nutty Professor to an evil witchdoctor. As ridiculous as that sounds, it seems to have an effect on a lot of people's opinions even as they continue to get sicker using modern medicine's standard interventions. Fortunately, the name-calling has no effect on me. While many news outlets have covered my books and articles with equal amounts of snarky ridicule and self-righteous outrage, what they never seem to offer is any solid evidence that convincingly contradicts what I've shared and my patients have experienced.

Words have power. Quite often in the press, specific words are chosen to send an implied message that taints as "crazy" not just the message the media is trying to suppress but the messenger himself. One particular reporter stated that an article I wrote for actress Gwyneth Paltrow's lifestyle website goop.com was based on a "long-discredited" theory.

To simply say the theory was *disproven* would be one thing. Lots of theories are tested and after evidence is viewed found to be ineffective. That's the way scientific research works. When a new drug or treatment fails in clinical trials, no one says the drug or intervention was "discredited." They simply say it was ineffective and move on. By saying the theory I based my viewpoint on was *discredited,* the reporter implied that my claim was illegitimate, even fraudulent, from the start. To be *discredited* is to have your credibility (trustworthiness) stripped from you and exposed as a liar. Yes, words matter, and by saying my viewpoint was *discredited* the reporter sent a very different message to the public than if he'd simply said my viewpoint was ineffective or outdated based on new research. Of course, there was no new research, and he accomplished what he set out to do with his word choice which was to attack my character and credibility.

My greatest fear with regard to the ridicule I've faced from working outside the medical box isn't the snide remarks from the media; it's that many sick patients will hear their words and never go on to read my work or the works of other physicians specializing in integrative healthcare and decide what's best for themselves. More healthcare information, especially evidence-based alternative viewpoints, means more choices, and more choices means more healthcare freedom for everyone so they can take an empowered role in their plan of care.

As this book draws to a close, let me remind you again that in 1847 Hungarian physician Ignaz Semmelweis had the audacity to suggest the absurd idea that something as simple as doctors washing their hands between patients while delivering babies could prevent thousands of mothers from dying from infection and puerperal fever. He was called a nutcase and "discredited" by the medical experts of his day too, and his career was ruined.

Just because the majority of people believe something doesn't make it true because the majority is often easily manipulated. New discoveries are never made by people from the majority but the outliers of society, the people willing to ask questions, challenge existing beliefs, and make great sacrifices. Truth is confirmed by evidence, and when it's your own body that experiences a miraculous healing there is no greater evidence of truth than that. For Semmelweis, the truth of his idea was confirmed when tens of thousands of women's lives were saved and they named a university after him.

Unconventional ideas *do* have something to offer in the way of disease prevention and saving lives, particularly where cancer is concerned. I owe my life to considering unconventional ideas during my battle with cancer nearly 30 years ago. It's my hope that patients everywhere will never relinquish their most powerful weapon in the fight to reclaim their health from cancer or any disease. It is the ability to educate themselves on all options available to them regardless of how unconventional they may seem to "the majority" then make a fully informed decision.

Back in 1987, I discovered anthropologist and behavioral scientist Robert Ardrey, author of *The Social Contract*. Ardrey explained how all animals have built-in alarm systems to alert them and their social group to danger. When one starling sounds an alarm, the entire flock takes to the air, flying in close formation and moving in unison often changing direction at odd angles and with sharp turns to confuse the oncoming predator. The visual overwhelm is enough to deter most birds of prey, including falcons.

The impulse to fall in formation with those around us and "do as the Romans do" is deeply ingrained in human survival instinct. The problem is that human beings are rarely in any mortal danger and yet regularly deny their personal opinions and desires, instead following the crowd to do what's more acceptable regardless of what they really think or want. They go along to get along.

Our prehistoric ancestors knew that to survive they had to work and stay together. Individual survival was dependent on group survival and remaining with others who could help find food, build shelter, and so on. To be separated from the group meant almost certain death. Even today we have a strong instinctual but unconscious association that equates separation from others with death. Although they may not realize it, it's the reason most people jump into fads and buy or wear something just because everyone else is doing it. Like a reflex, this unconscious behavior arises from the need to belong which is synonymous with the need to survive.

It's not easy to break with what everyone else is doing in medicine. I know what it's like to forge a new path while resisting cookie-cutter symptom management. It saddens me when physicians admire my practice and patient outcomes yet still reply with comments such as, "That would be *so* different for me. What if I lost the respect of my colleagues? What if patients left my practice?" or even worse "That's just not the way we do it at my clinic."

Of course, it isn't the way they do it. That's the whole purpose of blazing a new trail and trying to move medicine forward instead of flying in the same patterns all the time going nowhere. It's trusting that taking a new direction will confirm your new vision.

Unlike birds, human trailblazers hold onto the hope that we won't be pecked to death if we move out of formation. Yes, there will be humiliation and even intimidation to return to the fold. We'll be called pseudoscientists and snake oil salesmen. Even so, if our courage holds out and we can resist the unconscious drive to conform we just might end up changing the world even if, like so many others who died before their achievements were recognized, we don't live to see how our "crazy" ideas made life better. The masters that have come before us have proven this to be true. Progress is always seen as blasphemy before it's recognized as a blessing.

As a doctor, patient, or author, the fact remains that if one has the courage to leave the flock, the next time we look back we just might find everyone else following us. The choice is ours. Eagles fly alone but sheep flock together.

About the Author

Dr. Habib Sadeghi is the founder of Entelechy Medical & Dental Community Center in Agoura Hills, California and a clinical instructor of family medicine at Western University of Health Sciences. He is the author of *WITHIN: a spiritual awakening to love and weight loss* and *The Clarity Cleanse: 12 steps to finding renewed energy, spiritual fulfillment, and emotional healing*, as well as the publisher of the health and wellness journal, *MegaZEN*. In 2013, he founded the nonprofit organization, the Love Button Global Movement. To find out more about Dr. Sadeghi, visit BeingClarity.com.

Acknowledgments

Patti Britton, PhD, MPH, ACSE whose instruction and expertise allowed me to create effective interventions for couples with intimacy challenges.

Susan Stiritz, PhD, MSW for cultivating my interest in sexual health and whose research on culture and sexual practices deeply informs my work.

Debra Wickman, MD who profoundly changed my perception of women's healthcare and what it means to empower patients through understanding their own bodies.

Bibliography

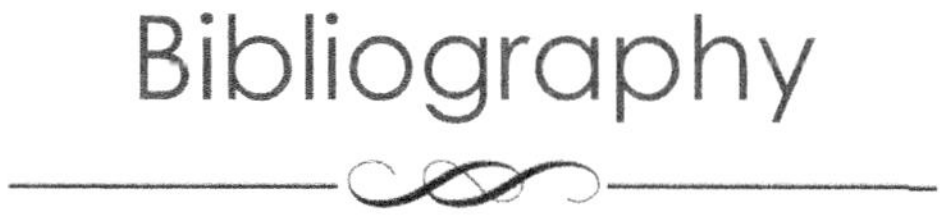

Introduction

[1] Kelland, Kelly, "Chronic Disease to Cost $47 Trillion by 2030: WEF", *Reuters*, (Sept. 18, 2011).
[2] This exploration included an eight-year mentorship with Jon Tabakin, PhD, FIPA, Training and Supervising Analyst at The Psychoanalytic Center of California.
[3] The late Dr. Morton Herskowitz, associate of psychotherapist Wilhelm Reich, was pivotal in helping me discover this mind-body connection. I was fortunate to have been Morton's protégé for many years, learning about orgonomy and the process of emotional armoring. The late Dr. Selma "Carol" Stoll, Dr. Herskowitz's student, was also central in my education. As a result of their combined accomplishments, I have committed myself to forwarding this work by facilitating its next evolution.
[4] Cassoni, P., Sapino, A., Marrocco, T., Chini, B., & Bussolati, G. (2004). Oxytocin and oxytocin receptors in cancer cells and proliferation. *Journal of Neuroendocrinology*, *16*(4), 362-364. https://doi.org/10.1111/j.0953-8194.2004.01165.x.
[5] Imanieh, M. H., Bagheri, F., & Alizadeh, A. M. (2014). Oxytocin has therapeutic effects on cancer, a hypothesis. *European Journal of Pharmacology*, *741*, 112-123. https://doi.org/10.1016/j.ejphar.2014.07.053.
[6] Xu, H., & Fu, S. (2017). The function of oxytocin: A potential biomarker for prostate cancer diagnosis and promoter of prostate cancer. *Oncotarget*, *8*(19), 31215-31226. https://doi.org/10.18632/oncotarget.16107.
[7] Lerman, B., & Harricharran, T. (2018). Oxytocin and cancer: An emerging link. *World Journal of Clinical Oncology*, *9*(5), 74-82. https://doi.org/10.5306/wjco.v9.i5.74.
[8] Fredrickson, B. L. (2013). *Love 2.0: Creating happiness and health in moments of connection*. Penguin.

Chapter 3

[1] Gray, J. (1992). *Men Are from Mars, Women Are from Venus: The classic guide to understanding the opposite sex* (1st ed.). HarperCollins.
[2] Deida, D. (1997). *It's a Guy Thing; An owner's manual for women* (1st ed.). Health Comm.
[3] Ingalhalikar, M., Smith, A., & Parker, D. (2013). Sex differences in the structural connectome of the human brain. *Proceedings of the National Academy of Sciences*, *111*(2), 823-828. https://doi.org/10.1073/pnas.1316909110.
[4] Ryali, S., Zhang, Y., & De los Angeles, C. (2024). Deep learning models reveal replicable, generalizable, and behaviorally relevant sex differences in human functional brain organization. *Proceedings of the National Academy of Sciences*, *121*(9). https://doi.org/10.1073/pnas.2310012121.

[5] Del Giudice, M., Booth, T., & Irwing, P. (2012). The distance between Mars and Venus: Measuring global sex differences in personality. *PLoS ONE*, *7*(1), e29265. https://doi.org/10.1371/journal.pone.0029265.

Chapter 5

[1] Fields, D. (2007, February/March). Sex and the Secret Nerve. *Scientific American Mind*, 21-27, https://www.scientificamerican.com/article/sex-and-the-secret-nerve/.

Chapter 6

[1] *BBC News | World | Americas | US couples seek separate bedrooms*. (2007, March 12). BBC News. https://news.bbc.co.uk/2/hi/americas/6441131.stm.
[2] Krasnow, I. (2012, July 4). *Separate bedrooms can steam up a marriage*. Huffington Post. https://www.huffingtonpost.com/iris-krasnow/separate-bedrooms-can-steam_b_1480448.html.
[3] Winter, K. (2014, June 30). *Couples spend longer in the bathroom together than they do at dinner*. DailyMail Online. https://www.dailymail.co.uk/femail/article-2674974/Is-bathroom-bonding-key-healthy-relationship-Couples-spend-time-washroom-dinner-table.html.
[4] Kalmus, H. (1955). The discrimination by the nose of the dog of individual human odours and in particular the odours of twins. *The British Journal of Animal Behaviour*, *3*(1), 25-31.
[5] Tebrich, S. (2011, August 4). *Human scent and its detection*. https://www.cia.gov/library/center-for-the-study-of-intelligence/kent-csi/vol5no2/html/v05i2a04p_0001.htm.
[6] Ibid.
[7] Porter, R., & Moore, J. (1981). Human Kin recognition by olfactory cues. *Physiology & Behavior*, *27*(3), 490-495. https://doi.org/10.1016/0031-9384(81)90337-1.
[8] Varendi, H., & Porter, R. H. (2001). Breast odour as the only maternal stimulus elicits crawling towards the odour source. *Acta Paediatrica*, *90*(4), 372-375. https://doi.org/10.1080/080352501119715.
[9] Kaitz, M., & Good, A. (1987). Mothers' recognition of their newborns by olfactory cues. *Developmental Psychobiology*, *20*(6), 587-591. https://doi.org/10.1002/dev.420200604.
[10] Savic, I., & Berglund, H. (2001). Smelling of odorous sex hormone-like compounds causes sex-differentiated hypothalamic activations in humans. *Neuron*, *31*(4), 661-668. https://doi.org/10.1016/s0896-6273(01)00390-7.
[11] Bensafi, M., Brown, W. M., & Tsutsui, T. (2003). Sex-steroid derived compounds induce sex-specific effects on autonomic nervous system function in humans. *Behavioral Neuroscience*, *117*(6), 1125-1134. https://doi.org/10.1037/0735-7044.117.6.1125.
[12] Wyart, C., & Webster, W. W. (2007). Smelling a single component of male sweat alters levels of cortisol in women. *The Journal of Neuroscience*, *27*(6), 1261-1265. https://doi.org/10.1523/jneurosci.4430-06.2007.

[13] Jacob, S., & McClintock, M. K. (2000). Psychological state and mood effects of Steroidal Chemosignals in women and men. *Hormones and Behavior*, *37*(1), 57-78. https://doi.org/10.1006/hbeh.1999.1559.
[14] Liebowitz, M. R., & Salman, E. (2014). Effect of an acute intranasal aerosol dose of PH94B on social and performance anxiety in women with social anxiety disorder. *American Journal of Psychiatry*, *171*(6), 675-682. https://doi.org/10.1176/appi.ajp.2014.12101342.
[15] Preti, G., & Wysocki, C. J. (2003). Male axillary extracts contain pheromones that affect pulsatile secretion of luteinizing hormone and mood in women Recipients. *Biology of Reproduction*, *68*(6), 2107-2113. https://doi.org/10.1095/biolreprod.102.008268.
[16] Doty, R. L., & Snyder, P. J. (1981). Endocrine, cardiovascular, and psychological correlates of olfactory sensitivity changes during the human menstrual cycle. *Journal of Comparative and Physiological Psychology*, *95*(1), 45-60. https://doi.org/10.1037/h0077755.
[17] Bensafi, M., & Brown, W. M. (2003). Sex-steroid derived compounds induce sex-specific effects on autonomic nervous system function in humans. *Behavioral Neuroscience*, *117*(6), 1125-1134. https://doi.org/10.1037/0735-7044.117.6.1125.
[18] Olsson, M., & Lundström, J. (2006). A putative female pheromone affects mood in men differently depending on social context. *European Review of Applied Psychology*, *56*(4), 279-284. https://doi.org/10.1016/j.erap.2005.09.010.
[19] Savic, I., & Berglund, H. (2001). Smelling of odorous sex hormone-like compounds causes sex-differentiated hypothalamic activations in humans. *Neuron*, *31*(4), 661-668. https://doi.org/10.1016/s0896-6273(01)00390-7.
[20] Savic, I., & Berglund, H. (2005). Brain response to putative pheromones in homosexual men. *Proceedings of the National Academy of Sciences*, *102*(20), 7356-7361. https://doi.org/10.1073/pnas.0407998102.
[21] Berglund, H., & Lindström, P. (2006). Brain response to putative pheromones in lesbian women. *Proceedings of the National Academy of Sciences*, *103*(21), 8269-8274. https://doi.org/10.1073/pnas.0600331103.
[22] Nicholson, B. (1984). Does kissing aid human bonding by semiochemical addiction? *British Journal of Dermatology*, *111*(5), 623-627. https://doi.org/10.1111/j.1365-2133.1984.tb06635.x
[23] Floyd, K., & Boren, J. P. (2009). Kissing in marital and cohabiting relationships: Effects on blood lipids, stress, and relationship satisfaction. *Western Journal of Communication*, *73*(2), 113-133. https://doi.org/10.1080/10570310902856071.
[24] Montagnier, L., & Aïssa, J. (2009). Electromagnetic signals are produced by aqueous nanostructures derived from bacterial DNA sequences. *Interdisciplinary Sciences: Computational Life Sciences*, *1*(2), 81-90. https://doi.org/10.1007/s12539-009-0036-7.

Chapter 8

[1] Miller, C. (2014, December 2). *The Divorce Surge is Over, But the Myth Lives On*. NYTimes.com. https://www.nytimes.com/2014/12/02/upshot/the-divorce-surge-is-over-but-the-myth-lives-on.html?_r=0.
[2] Glantz, J. (2017, February 3). *Couples Who've been married for 50 years share their secrets to staying in love*. EliteDaily.com. https://www.elitedaily.com/dating/couples-married-for-50-years-secrets/1776876.

[3] Ibid.
[4] O'Neill, J. (2015, October 15). *16 relationship secrets to learn from couples married for 50+ years*. Good Housekeeping. https://www.goodhousekeeping.com/life/relationships/g2837/secrets-to-50-years-marriage/.
[5] Ibid.
[6] Ibid.
[7] Ibid.
[8] Bayless, K. (2015, December 14). *8 things people married for 50 years do.* Prevention.com. https://www.prevention.com/sex/a20491380/8-things-people-married-for-50-years-do/.
[9] Ibid.
[10] Glantz, J. (2017, February 3). *Couples Who've been married for 50 years share their secrets to staying in love.* EliteDaily.com. https://www.elitedaily.com/dating/couples-married-for-50-years-secrets/1776876.

Chapter 11

[1] Bieber, C., & Johnaon, J. (2023, August 8). *Revealing divorce statistics in 2023.* Forbes Advisor. https://www.forbes.com/advisor/legal/divorce/divorce-statistics/.
[2] Kaplan, H., & Hill, K. (2000). A theory of human life history evolution: Diet, intelligence, and longevity. *Evolutionary Anthropology: Issues, News, and Reviews*, *9*(4), 156-185. https://doi.org/10.1002/1520-6505(2000)9:4<156::aid-evan5>3.0.co;2-7.
[3] *FastStats Life Expectancy*. (2024, May 2). Centers for Disease Control and Prevention. https://www.cdc.gov/nchs/fastats/life-expectancy.htm.
[4] *Conscious uncoupling.* (2024, July 27). Wikipedia, the free encyclopedia. Retrieved August 11, 2024, from https://en.wikipedia.org/wiki/Conscious_uncoupling.

Chapter 12

[1] Female Orgasms: myths & facts. The Society of Obstetricians and Gynecologists of Canada, https://sogc.org/publications/female-orgasms-myths-and-facts/.
[2] Thacker, H. (2014, June 4). *There's Help for Women Who Can't Achieve Orgasm.* Cleveland Clinic Health Essentials. https://health.clevelandclinic.org/2014/06/help-for-women-who-cant-easily-orgasm.
[3] Donaldson-James, S. (2009, September 3). *Female orgasm may be tied to 'Rule of thumb'.* ABC News. https://abcnews.go.com/Health/ReproductiveHealth/sex-study-female-orgasm-eludes-majority-women/story?id=8485289.
[4] Thomas, L. (2011, November 11). *Help! I can't have an orgasm.* Psychology Today. https://www.psychologytoday.com/us/blog/save-your-sex-life/201111/help-i-cant-have-orgasm.
[5] Castleman, M. (2016, February 1). *Why so many women don't have orgasms.* Psychology Today. https://www.psychologytoday.com/us/blog/all-about-sex/201602/why-so-many-women-don-t-have-orgasms.

[6] Lloyd, E. A. (2006). *The case of the female orgasm: Bias in the science of evolution.* Harvard University Press.
[7] Galinsky, A. M. (2011). Sexual touching and difficulties with sexual arousal and orgasm among U.S. older adults. *Archives of Sexual Behavior*, *41*(4), 875-890. https://doi.org/10.1007/s10508-011-9873-7.
[8] Corty, E. W., & Guardiani, J. M. (2008). Canadian and American sex therapists' perceptions of normal and abnormal ejaculatory Latencies: How long should intercourse last? *The Journal of Sexual Medicine*, *5*(5), 1251-1256. https://doi.org/10.1111/j.1743-6109.2008.00797.x.

Chapter 13

[1] *FastStats Infertility*. (2023, February 23). Centers for Disease Control and Prevention. https://www.cdc.gov/nchs/fastats/infertility.htm.
[2] Liu, J., & Yuan, W. (2023). Thallium pollution from the lithium industry calls for urgent international action on regulations. *Environmental Science & Technology*, *57*(48), 19099-19101. https://doi.org/10.1021/acs.est.3c08267.
[3] Liang, C., & Luo, G. (2022). Environmental thallium exposure and the risk of early embryonic arrest among women undergoing in vitro fertilization: Thallium exposure and polymorphisms of mtDNA gene interaction and potential cause exploring. *Environmental Science and Pollution Research*, *29*(41), 62648-62661. https://doi.org/10.1007/s11356-022-19978-2.
[4] López-Botella, A., & Velasco, I. (2021). Impact of heavy metals on human male fertility—An overview. *Antioxidants*, *10*(9), 1473. https://doi.org/10.3390/antiox10091473.
[5] Bade, T., & Kats, A. (2011). Expression of Prostaglandin E Synthases in Periodontitis. https://doi.org/10.1016/j.ajpath.2010.12.048.

Chapter 14

[1] Welch, H. G., & Black, W. C. (1997). Using autopsy series to estimate the disease "Reservoir" for ductal carcinoma in situ of the breast: How much more breast cancer can we find? *Annals of Internal Medicine*, *127*(11), 1023-1028. https://doi.org/10.7326/0003-4819-127-11-199712010-00014.
[2] Nielsen, M., & Thomsen, J. (1987). Breast cancer and atypia among young and middle-aged women: A study of 110 medicolegal autopsies. *British Journal of Cancer*, *56*(6), 814-819. https://doi.org/10.1038/bjc.1987.296.
[3] Northrup, C. (2012). *The wisdom of menopause: Creating physical and emotional health during the change*. Hay House, pg. 528.
[4] Bleyer, A., & Welch, H. G. (2012). Effect of three decades of screening mammography on breast-cancer incidence. *New England Journal of Medicine*, *367*(21), 1998-2005. https://doi.org/10.1056/nejmoa1206809.
[5] Moody-Ayers, S. Y., & Wells, C. K. (2000). "Benign" Tumors and "Early detection" in mammography-screened patients of a natural cohort with breast cancer. *Archives of Internal Medicine*, *160*(8), 1109. https://doi.org/10.1001/archinte.160.8.1109.

[6] *American Cancer Society Recommendations for the Early Detection of Breast Cancer.* (2024, July 6). American Cancer Society. https://www.cancer.org/cancer/news/news/american-cancer-society-releases-new-breast-cancer-guidelines.
[7] *Limitations of mammograms.* (2022, January 14). American Cancer Society. https://www.cancer.org/cancer/types/breast-cancer/screening-tests-and-early-detection/mammograms/limitations-of-mammograms.html.
[8] *Breast cancer screening.* (2023, June 26). National Cancer Institute. https://www.cancer.gov/types/breast/patient/breast-screening-pdq.
[9] Elmore, J. G., & Barton, M. B. (1998). Ten-year risk of false positive screening mammograms and clinical breast examinations. *New England Journal of Medicine, 338*(16), 1089-1096. https://doi.org/10.1056/nejm199804163381601.
[10] *Breast cancer screening.* (2023, June 26). National Cancer Institute. https://www.cancer.gov/types/breast/patient/breast-screening-pdq.
[11] *Mammograms.* (2023, February 21). National Cancer Institute. https://www.cancer.gov/types/breast/mammograms-fact-sheet.
[12] Gøtzsche, P. C., & Olsen, O. (2000). Is screening for breast cancer with mammography justifiable? *The Lancet, 355*(9198), 129-134. https://doi.org/10.1016/s0140-6736(99)06065-1
[13] *Breast cancer screening.* (2023, June 26). National Cancer Institute. https://www.cancer.gov/types/breast/patient/breast-screening-pdq.
[14] *Radiation risk from medical imaging.* (2021, September 30). Harvard Health. https://www.health.harvard.edu/cancer/radiation-risk-from-medical-imaging.
[15] Pauwels, E. K., & Foray, N. (2015). Breast cancer induced by X-ray mammography screening? A review based on recent understanding of low-dose radiobiology. *Medical Principles and Practice, 25*(2), 101-109. https://doi.org/10.1159/000442442.
[16] Mambou, S. J., & Maresova, P. (2018). Breast cancer detection using infrared thermal imaging and a deep learning model. *Sensors, 18*(9), 2799. https://doi.org/10.3390/s18092799.
[17] Parisky, Y. R., & Sardi, A. (2003). Efficacy of computerized infrared imaging analysis to evaluate Mammographically suspicious lesions. *American Journal of Roentgenology, 180*(1), 263-269. https://doi.org/10.2214/ajr.180.1.1800263.
[18] Morales-Cervantes, A., & Kolosovas-Machuca, E. S. (2018). An automated method for the evaluation of breast cancer using infrared thermography. *EXCLI Journal, 17*(1), 989–998. https://doi.org/0.17179/excli2018-1735.
[19] *What is breast thermography.* (2003). International Academy of Thermology. https://www.iact-org.org/patients/breastthermography/what-is-breast-therm.html.

Chapter 15

[1] Eunjung Cha, A. (2018, January 27). *The Struggle to Conceive with Frozen Eggs*. The Washington Post. https://www.washingtonpost.com/news/national/wp/2018/01/27/feature/she-championed-the-idea-that-freezing-your-eggs-would-free-your-career-but-things-didnt-quite-work-out/?utm_term=.a7ad08416826.

---

[2] Tsigoinos, P. M. (2014, October 27). *Here are the unspoken egg-freezing facts*. WIRED. https://www.wired.com/story/egg-freezing-facts/.
[3] Miles, K., & Hackman, S. (2023, November 28). *What are your chances of getting pregnant at different ages?* BabyCenter. https://www.babycenter.com/getting-pregnant/preparing-for-pregnancy/chart-the-effect-of-age-on-fertility_6155.
[4] Faraday, J. (2023, August 10). *The guide to egg freezing costs in the US*. FamilyEducation. https://www.familyeducation.com/pregnancy/trying-to-conceive/the-guide-to-egg-freezing-costs-in-the-us.
[5] Cil, A. P., Bang, H., & Oktay, K. (2013). Age-specific probability of live birth with oocyte cryopreservation: An individual patient data meta-analysis. *Fertility and Sterility*, *100*(2), 492-499.e3. https://doi.org/10.1016/j.fertnstert.2013.04.023.
[6] *American Society for Reproductive Medicine Fact Sheet: Can I freeze my eggs to use later if I'm not sick?* (2014). FertilityAnswers.com. https://www.fertilityanswers.com/wp-content/uploads/2016/04/can-i-freeze-my-eggs-to-use-later-if-i-m-not-sick.pdf.
[7] Schuman, L., & Copperman, K. (2011). Trends in age in non-medical oocyte cryopreservation. *Fertility & Sterility*, *96*(3), 112-125. https://doi.org/10.1016/j.fertnstert.2011.07.596.
[8] Motluk, A. (2011). Growth of egg freezing blurs 'experimental' label. *Nature*, *476*(7361), 382-383. https://doi.org/10.1038/476382a.
[9] Rudick, B., & Opper, N. (2010). The status of oocyte cryopreservation in the United States. *Fertility and Sterility*, *94*(7), 2642-2646. https://doi.org/10.1016/j.fertnstert.2010.04.079.
[10] Gafson, I. (2014, October 17). *The facts don't lie: We haven't cracked egg freezing. Not even close*. The Telegraph. https://www.telegraph.co.uk/women/womens-life/11169420/Facebook-egg-freezing-The-facts-dont-lie-We-havent-cracked-egg-freezing.-Not-even-close.html.
[11] Goldman, R., & Racowsky, C. (2017). Predicting the likelihood of live birth for elective oocyte cryopreservation: A counseling tool for physicians and patients. *Human Reproduction*, *32*(4), 853-859. https://doi.org/10.1093/humrep/dex008.
[12] Kakkar, P., & Geary, J. (2023). Outcomes of social egg freezing: A cohort study and a comprehensive literature review. *Journal of Clinical Medicine*, *12*(13), 4182. https://doi.org/10.3390/jcm12134182.
[13] Eunjung Cha, A. (2018, January 27). *The Struggle to Conceive with Frozen Eggs*. The Washington Post. https://www.washingtonpost.com/news/national/wp/2018/01/27/feature/she-championed-the-idea-that-freezing-your-eggs-would-free-your-career-but-things-didnt-quite-work-out/?utm_term=.a7ad08416826.
[14] Darnovsky, M. (2014, October 15). *Egg freezing poses health risks to women*. Center for Genetics and Society. https://www.geneticsandsociety.org/press-statement/egg-freezing-poses-health-risks-women.
[15] Feinberg, R. "Elective Egg Freezing: 10 Thoughts from an REI", Obgyn.net, (Oct. 17, 2014), https://www.obgyn.net/ivf/elective-egg-freezing-10-thoughts-rei.
[16] Greenwood, E. A., & Pasch, L. A. (2018). To freeze or not to freeze: Decision regret and satisfaction following elective oocyte cryopreservation. *Fertility and Sterility*, *109*(6), 1097-1104.e1. https://doi.org/10.1016/j.fertnstert.2018.02.127.

[17] Eunjung Cha, A. (2018, January 27). *The Struggle to Conceive with Frozen Eggs*. The Washington Post. https://www.washingtonpost.com/news/national/wp/2018/01/27/feature/she-championed-the-idea-that-freezing-your-eggs-would-free-your-career-but-things-didnt-quite-work-out/?utm_term=.a7ad08416826.

[18] ASRM Office of Public Affairs. (2012, October 22). *Fertility Experts Issue New Report on Egg Freezing; ASRM Lifts "Experimental" Label from Technique.* TXfertility.com. https://txfertility.com/wp-content/uploads/2014/01/ASRMeggfreezerelease.pdf.

[19] Practice Committees of the American Society for Reproductive Medicine and the Society for Assisted Reproductive Technology. (2013). Mature oocyte cryopreservation: A guideline. *Fertility and Sterility*, *99*(1), 37-43. https://doi.org/10.1016/j.fertnstert.2012.09.028.

[20] American College of Obstetricians and Gynecologists. (2014). Committee opinion No. 584. *Obstetrics and Gynecology*, *123*(1), 221-222. https://doi.org/10.1097/01.aog.0000441355.66434.6d

[21] Darnovsky, M. (2014, October 15). *Egg freezing poses health risks to women.* Center for Genetics and Society. https://www.geneticsandsociety.org/press-statement/egg-freezing-poses-health-risks-women.

[22] Sydell, L. (2014, October 17). *Silicon Valley companies add new benefit for women: Egg-freezing*. NPR. https://www.npr.org/sections/alltechconsidered/2014/10/17/356765423/silicon-valley-companies-add-new-benefit-for-women-egg-freezing.

[23] Walden, R. (2014, October 28). *Why corporate promotion of egg freezing isn't a "Benefit" to all women.* Ourbodiesourselves.org. https://www.ourbodiesourselves.org/blog/apple-facebook-cover-egg-freezing/.

Chapter 16

[1] Agency for Healthcare Research and Quality. (n.d.). *Safety of Vaccines Used for Routine Immunization in the United States: Evidence Report / Technology Assessment Number 215*. National Institutes of Health. https://www.ncbi.nlm.nih.gov/books/NBK230053/pdf/Bookshelf_NBK230053.pdf

[2] The National Academy of Sciences, Engineering, and Medicine. (1991). *Adverse Effects of Pertussis and Rubella Vaccines*. The National Academies Press. https://www.nap.edu/read/1815/chapter/2.

[3] Hooker, B. S. (2014). Measles-mumps-rubella vaccination timing and autism among young African American boys: A reanalysis of CDC data. *Translational Neurodegeneration*, *3*(16). https://doi.org/10.1186/2047-9158-3-16.

[4] Attkisson, A. (2023, July 16). *Dr. Andrew Zimmerman's full Affidavit on alleged link between vaccines and autism that U.S. govt. covered up*. SharylAttkisson.com. https://sharylattkisson.com/2019/01/dr-andrew-zimmermans-full-affidavit-on-alleged-link-between-vaccines-and-autism-that-u-s-govt-covered-up.

[5] Blaxill, M. F. (2004). What's going on? The question of time trends in autism. *Public Health Reports*, *119*(6), 536-551. https://doi.org/10.1016/j.phr.2004.09.003.

[6] Centers for Disease Control and Prevention. (2024, February 22). *Data and statistics on autism spectrum disorder*. Autism Spectrum Disorder (ASD). https://www.cdc.gov/autism/data-research/index.html.
[7] Centers for Disease Control and Prevention. (2022, January 25). *Autism and vaccines*. https://www.cdc.gov/vaccinesafety/concerns/autism.html.
[8] Kennedy, R. F. (2019, August 15). *Americans can handle an open discussion on vaccines—RFK Jr. Responds to criticism from his family*. Children's Health Defense. https://childrenshealthdefense.org/news/americans-can-handle-an-open-discussion-on-vaccines-rfk-jr-responds-to-criticism-from-his-family/.
[9] Mogensen, S. W., & Andersen, A. (2017). The introduction of diphtheria-tetanus-Pertussis and oral polio vaccine among young infants in an urban African community: A natural experiment. *EBioMedicine*, *17*, 192-198. https://doi.org/10.1016/j.ebiom.2017.01.041.
[10] Kennedy, R. F. (2019, August 15). *Americans can handle an open discussion on vaccines—RFK Jr. Responds to criticism from his family*. Children's Health Defense. https://childrenshealthdefense.org/news/americans-can-handle-an-open-discussion-on-vaccines-rfk-jr-responds-to-criticism-from-his-family/.
[11] Legal Information Institute Cornell Law School. (2022, July 6). *15 U.S. code § 3710c - Distribution of royalties received by federal agencies*. LII / Legal Information Institute. https://www.law.cornell.edu/uscode/text/15/3710c.
[12] Mikulic, M. (2022, July 27). *Global Vaccine Market Revenues from 2014 to 2020*. Statista. https://www.statista.com/statistics/265102/revenues-in-the-global-vaccine-market/.
[13] Almashat, S., & Lang, R. (2018). *Twenty-Seven Years of Pharmaceutical Industry Criminal and Civil Penalties: 1991 Through 2017*. Public Citizen. https://www.citizen.org/wp-content/uploads/2408.pdf.
[14] Park, A. (2020, December 11). *The First Authorized COVID-19 Vaccine in the U.S. Has Arrived*. TIME. https://time.com/5920134/first-authorized-covid-19-vaccine-us/.
[15] Lance, R. (2021, June 29). *How COVID-19 vaccines were made so quickly without cutting corners*. Science News. https://www.sciencenews.org/article/covid-coronavirus-vaccine-development-speed.
[16] Institute of Medicine of the National Academies. (2013). *The Childhood Immunization Schedule and Safety: Stakeholder Concerns, Scientific Evidence, and Future Studies The Childhood Immunization Schedule and Safety Stakeholder Concerns, Scientific Evidence, and Future Studies*. National Academies. https://www.nap.edu/catalog/13563/the-childhood-immunization-schedule-and-safety-stakeholder-concerns-scientific-evidence.
[17] Van Cleave, J. (2010). Dynamics of obesity and chronic health conditions among children and youth. *JAMA*, *303*(7), 623-630. https://doi.org/10.1001/jama.2010.104.
[18] Bethell, C. D., & Kogan, M. D. (2011). A national and state profile of leading health problems and health care quality for US children: Key insurance disparities and across-state variations. *Academic Pediatrics*, *11*(3), S22-S33. https://doi.org/10.1016/j.acap.2010.08.011.
[19] Miller, L., & Lu, W. (2019, February 24). *These Are the World's Healthiest Nations*. Bloomberg . https://www.bloomberg.com/news/articles/2019-02-24/spain-tops-italy-as-world-s-healthiest-nation-while-u-s-slips.

[20] Trimble, M. (2018, January 11). *U.S. Kids More Likely to Die Than Kids in 19 Other Nations*. US News & World Report. https://www.usnews.com/news/best-countries/articles/2018-01-11/us-has-highest-child-mortality-rate-of-20-rich-countries.
[21] Bigtree, D. (2018, December 31). Informed Consent Action Network. *HHS Vaccine Safety Responsibilities and Notice Pursuant to 42 U.S.C. § 300aa-31*. Children's Health Defense. https://childrenshealthdefense.org/wp-content/uploads/ican-reply-december-31-2018.pdf.
[22] Institute of Medicine Vaccine Safety Committee. (1991). *Adverse Effects of Pertussis and Rubella Vaccines: A Report of the Committee to Review the Adverse Consequences of Pertussis and Rubella Vaccines* (1st ed.). National Academies Press. https://doi.org/10.17226/1815.
[23] Institute of Medicine Vaccine Safety Committee. (1994). *Adverse Events Associated with Childhood Vaccines: Evidence Bearing on Causality* (1st ed.). National Academies Press. https://doi.org/10.17226/2138.
[24] Health Resources and Services Administration. (2024, July 1). *National Vaccine Injury Compensation Program Data Report*. HSRA.gov. https://www.hrsa.gov/sites/default/files/hrsa/vicp/vicp-stats-07-01-24.pdf.
[25] Centers for Disease Control and Prevention. (searched 2024, July 15). *The Vaccine Adverse Event Reporting System*. CDC. https://wonder.cdc.gov/controller/datarequest/D8.
[26] Lazarus, R. (2010). *Grant Final Report, Electronic Support for Public Health–Vaccine Adverse Event Reporting System (ESP:VAERS)* (Grant ID: R18 HS 017045). Agency for Healthcare Research and Quality. https://digital.ahrq.gov/sites/default/files/docs/publication/r18hs017045-lazarus-final-report-2011.pdf.
[27] Picchi, A. (2016, March 11). *Drug ads: $5.2 billion annually -- and rising*. CBS News - Breaking news, 24/7 live streaming news & top stories. https://www.cbsnews.com/news/drug-ads-5-2-billion-annually-and-rising/.
[28] Centers for Disease Control and Prevention. (2017, July). *Genital HPV infection – CDC fact sheet*. CDC.gov. https://stacks.cdc.gov/view/cdc/130186.
[29] Centers for Disease Control and Prevention. (2024, June 13). *Cervical Cancer Statistics*. CDC.gov. https://www.cdc.gov/cervical-cancer/statistics/index.html.
[30] Centers for Disease Control and Prevention. (2023, November 14). *Cancers Linked With HPV Each Year*. CDC.gov. https://www.cdc.gov/cancer/hpv/cases.htm.
[31] Molano, M. (2003). Determinants of clearance of human papillomavirus infections in colombian women with normal cytology: A population-based, 5-Year follow-up study. *American Journal of Epidemiology*, *158*(5), 486-494. https://doi.org/10.1093/aje/kwg171.
[32] Franco, E., & Villa, L. (1999). Epidemiology of acquisition and clearance of cervical human papillomavirus infection in women from a high-risk area for cervical cancer. *The Journal of Infectious Diseases*, *180*(5), 1415-1423. https://doi.org/10.1086/315086.
[33] Ho, G. Y., & Burk, R. D. (1995). Persistent genital human papillomavirus infection as a risk factor for persistent cervical dysplasia. *JNCI Journal of the National Cancer Institute*, *87*(18), 1365-1371. https://doi.org/10.1093/jnci/87.18.1365.
[34] Thompson, Z. (2019, August 8). *Does HPV go away on its own or does it stick around forever?*. SELF. https://www.self.com/story/does-hpv-go-away.
[35] Centers for Disease Control and Prevention. (2022, March 9). *Manual for the Surveillance of Vaccine-Preventable Diseases: Chapter 5: Human Papillomavirus*. CDC.gov. https://www.cdc.gov/vaccines/pubs/surv-manual/chpt05-hpv.html.

[36] Winer, R., & Hughes, J. (2006). Condom use and the risk of genital human papillomavirus infection in young women. *NEJM, 354*(25), 2645-2654. https://doi.org/10.1056/NEJMoa053284.
[37] Centers for Disease Control and Prevention. (searched 2024, July 15). *The Vaccine Adverse Event Reporting System*. CDC. https://wonder.cdc.gov/controller/datarequest/D8.
[38] Little, D. T., & Ward, H. R. (2014). Adolescent premature ovarian insufficiency following human papillomavirus vaccination. *Journal of Investigative Medicine High Impact Case Reports, 2*(4), 232470961455612. https://doi.org/10.1177/2324709614556129.
[39] Little, D. T., & Ward, H. R. (2012). Premature ovarian failure 3 years after menarche in a 16-year-old girl following human papillomavirus vaccination. *BMJ Case Reports, 45*(7), bcr2012006879. https://doi.org/10.1136/bcr-2012-006879.
[40] Wetzstein, C. (2013, November 11). *HPV Vaccine Cited in Infertility Case*. The Washington Times. https://www.washingtontimes.com/news/2013/nov/11/hpv-vaccine-cited-in-infertility-case.
[41] DeLong, D. (2016, May 19). *Judge dismisses lawsuit: Wisconsin sisters say Gardasil vaccine caused their premature ovarian failure*. FOX6 News Milwaukee. https://fox6now.com/2016/05/19/judge-dismisses-lawsuit-wisconsin-sisters-say-gardasil-vaccine-caused-their-premature-ovarian-failure.
[42] *Cervarix vaccine issues trigger health notice*. (2013, June 15). The Japan Times. https://www.japantimes.co.jp/news/2013/06/15/national/cervix-vaccine-issues-trigger-health-notice/#.VwiG1BMrL-Z.
[43] DeLong, G. (n.d.). A lowered probability of pregnancy in females in the USA aged 25-29 who received a human papillomavirus vaccine injection. *Journal of Toxicology and Environmental Health, 81*(14), 661-674. https://doi.org/10.1080/15287394.2018.1477640.
[44] Editors. (2018). Retracted article: [A lowered probability of pregnancy in females in the USA aged 25–29 who received a human papillomavirus vaccine injection]. *Journal of Toxicology and Environmental Health, Part A, 81*(14), 661–674. https://doi.org/10.1080/15287394.2018.1477640.
[45] DeLong, G. (2019). Letters to the editor; Response to: A possible spurious correlation between human papillomavirus vaccination introduction and birth rate change in the United States. *Human Vaccines & Immunotherapeutics, 15*(10), 2503-2504. https://doi.org/10.1080/21645515.2019.1622977.
[46] Field, S. (2016, January). *Press Release: New Concerns About the Human Papilloma Virus Vaccine*. https://www.acpeds.org/the-college-speaks/position-statements/health-issues/new-concerns-about-the-human-papillomavirus-vaccine.
[47] Dirnhofer, S., & Klieber, R. (1993). Functional and immunological relevance of the COOH-terminal extension of human chorionic gonadotropin beta: Implications for the WHO birth control vaccine. *The FASEB Journal, 7*(14), 1381-1385. https://doi.org/10.1096/fasebj.7.14.7693535.
[48] Aiken, R. J., & Paterson, M. (1993). Contraceptive vaccines. *British Medical Bulletin, 49*(1), 88-99. https://doi.org/10.1093/oxfordjournals.bmb.a072608.
[49] PubMed, Best Matches for Contraceptive Vaccines, https://www.ncbi.nlm.nih.gov/pubmed?orig_db=PubMed&cmd=Search&TransSchema=title&term=contraceptive+vaccine.

[50] Talwar, G. P., & Raghupathy, R. (1989). Anti-fertility vaccines. *Vaccine*, *7*(2), 97-101. https://doi.org/10.1016/0264-410x(89)90043-1.
[51] Wetherbe, S. (2014, November 6). *'A mass sterilization exercise': Kenyan doctors find anti-fertility agent in UN tetanus vaccine*. LifeSite. https://www.lifesitenews.com/news/a-mass-sterilization-exercise-kenyan-doctors-find-anti-fertility-agent-in-u.
[52] Hoffman. (2008, August 14). *Massive Brazilian Vaccination Raises Suspicions of Covert Sterilization Program*. LifeSite. https://www.lifesitenews.com/news/massive-brazilian-vaccination-raises-suspicions-of-covert-sterilization-pro.
[53] Gajdová, M., & Jakubovsky, J. (1993). Delayed effects of neonatal exposure to tween 80 on female reproductive organs in rats. *Food and Chemical Toxicology*, *31*(3), 183-190. https://doi.org/10.1016/0278-6915(93)90092-d.
[54] *Fluzone high-dose: Package insert*. (2024, March 18). Drugs.com. https://www.drugs.com/pro/fluzone-high-dose.html.
[55] Delepine, N. (2019, January 31). *Paradoxical effect of anti-hpv vaccine GARDASIL on cervical cancer rate – Docteur Nicole Delépine*. https://docteur.nicoledelepine.fr/. https://docteur.nicoledelepine.fr/paradoxical-effect-of-anti-hpv-vaccine-gardasil-on-cervical-cancer-rate/#_ftnref1.
[56] Ibid.
[57] National Cancer Institute. (2024). *Cancer Stat Facts: Cervical Cancer*. cancer.gov. https://seer.cancer.gov/statfacts/html/cervix.html.
[58] Andersson, L. (2018). Increased incidence of cervical cancer in Sweden: Possible link with HPV vaccination. *Indian Journal of Medical Ethics*, 1-5. https://doi.org/10.20529/ijme.2018.037.
[59] Editors of the Indian Journal of Medical Ethics. (2018). RETRACTION: Increased incidence of cervical cancer in Sweden: Possible link with HPV vaccination. *Indian Journal of Medical Ethics*, *3*(3), 246. https://doi.org/10.20529/IJME.2018.057.
[60] Moberly, T. (2017). UK doctors re-examine case for mandatory vaccination. *BMJ*, *358*. https://doi.org/10.1136/bmj.j3414.
[61] Jankowska, A., & Gunderson, S. I. (2008). Reduction of human chorionic gonadotropin beta subunit expression by modified U1 snRNA caused apoptosis in cervical cancer cells. *Molecular Cancer*, *7*(1), 26. https://doi.org/10.1186/1476-4598-7-26.
[62] Naz, R. K., & Gupta, S. K. (2005). Recent advances in contraceptive vaccine development: A mini-review. *Human Reproduction*, *20*(12), 3271-3283 https://doi.org/10.1093/humrep/dei256
[63] Hinks, S. (2018). Rapid response to: HPV vaccines are effective and safe and work best in young women, review finds. *British Medical Journal*, *361*. https://www.bmj.com/content/361/bmj.k2059/rr-6.
[64] Walia, A. (2019, April 5). *Robert F. Kennedy Jr explains the dangers of the HPV*. LewRockwell.com. https://www.lewrockwell.com/2019/04/no_author/robert-f-kennedy-jr-explains-dangers-of-the-hpv-how-it-could-give-you-cancer/.

Chapter 17

[1] *About the Menopause Research & Equity Act of 2023*. (2023). Let's Talk Menopause.org. https://www.letstalkmenopause.org/advocacy.

[2] Northrup, C. (2001). *The wisdom of menopause: Creating physical and emotional health and healing during the change* (1st ed.). pg. 120. Bantam Books.

[3] Smith, D. C., & Prentice, R. (1975). Association of exogenous estrogen and endometrial carcinoma. *New England Journal of Medicine*, *293*(23), 1164-1167. https://doi.org/10.1056/nejm197512042932302.

[4] Grodstein, F., & Manson, J. E. (2006). Hormone therapy and coronary heart disease: The role of time since menopause and age at hormone initiation. *Journal of Women's Health*, *15*(1), 35-44. https://doi.org/10.1089/jwh.2006.15.35.

[5] Grodstein, F., & Manson, J. E. (2000). A prospective, observational study of postmenopausal hormone therapy and primary prevention of cardiovascular disease. *Annals of Internal Medicine*, *133*(12), 933. https://doi.org/10.7326/0003-4819-133-12-200012190-00008.

[6] Hulley, S. (1998). Randomized trial of estrogen plus progestin for secondary prevention of coronary heart disease in postmenopausal women. *JAMA*, *280*(7), 605-613. https://doi.org/10.1001/jama.280.7.605.

[7] Chlebowski, R. T., & Anderson, G. L. (2010). Estrogen plus progestin and breast cancer incidence and mortality in postmenopausal women. *Journal of the American Medical Association*, *304*(15), 1684-1692.

[8] Urban, P. (2023). *Deadliest Cancers in the U.S. in 2023: Lung cancer tops list, taking an estimated 350 lives each day, according to American Cancer Society report.* AARP.com. https://www.aarp.org/health/conditions-treatments/info-2023/deadliest-cancers-for-men-and-women.html.

[9] Bhavnani, B. R. (1998). Pharmacokinetics and pharmacodynamics of conjugated equine estrogens: Chemistry and metabolism. *Experimental Biology and Medicine*, *217*(1), 6-16. https://doi.org/10.3181/00379727-217-44199.

[10] Shen, L., & Qiu, S. (1998). Alkylation of 2'-Deoxynucleosides and DNA by the Premarin metabolite 4-Hydroxyequilenin Semiquinone radical. *Chemical Research in Toxicology*, *11*(2), 94-101. https://doi.org/10.1021/tx970181r.

[11] Zhang, F., & Chen, Y. (1999). The major metabolite of Equilin, 4-Hydroxyequilin, Autoxidizes to an *o*-quinone which isomerizes to the potent cytotoxin 4-Hydroxyequilenin-<i>o</i>-quinone. *Chemical Research in Toxicology*, *12*(2), 204-213. https://doi.org/10.1021/tx980217v.

[12] Hulley, S. (1998). Randomized trial of estrogen plus progestin for secondary prevention of coronary heart disease in postmenopausal women. *JAMA*, *280*(7), 605-613. https://doi.org/10.1001/jama.280.7.605.

[13] *Anabolic Steroids: types, uses and risks: Methyltestosterone*. (2024). Steroids.com. https://www.steroid.com/Methyltestosterone.php.

[14] Hodis, H. N., & Mack, W. J. (2014). Testing the menopausal hormone therapy timing hypothesis: the Early Vs Late Intervention Trial with Estradiol. *Circulation*, *130*, A13283.. https://www.ahajournals.org/doi/10.1161/circ.130.suppl_2.13283.

[15] Karim, R., & Xu, W. (2022). Effect of menopausal hormone therapy on arterial wall echomorphology: Results from the early versus late intervention trial with Estradiol (ELITE). *Maturitas*, *162*, 15-22. https://doi.org/10.1016/j.maturitas.2022.02.007.
[16] Tsagkas, V. (2012, October 3). *Hormone Therapy Has Many Favorable Effects in Newly Menopausal Women: Initial Findings of the Kronos Early Estrogen Prevention Study (KEEPS)*. pharmastar.it.
https://www.pharmastar.it/binary_files/allegati/general_release_67741.pdf.
[17] Miller, V. M., & Taylor, H. S. (2020). Lessons from KEEPS: The Kronos early estrogen prevention study. *Climacteric*, *24*(2), 139-145.
https://doi.org/10.1080/13697137.2020.1804545.
[18] National Institute on Aging. (2022, May 6). *Research Highlights: Research explores the impact of menopause on women's health and aging*. NIA.NIH.gov.
https://www.nia.nih.gov/news/research-explores-impact-menopause-womens-health-and-aging.

Chapter 18

[1] Epstein, A. (Director). (2012). *The Business of Being Born* [DVD]. New Line Home Video.
[2] Ehrenthal, D. B., & Jiang, X. (2010). Labor induction and the risk of a cesarean delivery among nulliparous women at term. *Obstetrics & Gynecology*, *116*(1), 35-42.
https://doi.org/10.1097/aog.0b013e3181e10c5c.
[3] Menacker, F., & Hamilton, B. E. (2010). Recent trends in cesarean delivery in the United States. *NCHS Data Brief*, *35*, 1-8. https://doi.org/10.1037/e665412010-001.
[4] Hamilton, B., & Martin, J. (2024, April). *Vital Statistics Rapid Release, Births: Provisional Data for 2023, Report No. 35*. CDC.gov.
https://www.cdc.gov/nchs/data/vsrr/vsrr035.pdf.
[5] Kuklina, E. V., & Meikle, S. F. (2009). Severe obstetric morbidity in the United States: 1998–2005. *Obstetrics & Gynecology*, *113*(2, Part 1), 293-299.
https://doi.org/10.1097/aog.0b013e3181954e5b.
[6] Russo, C. A., & Wier, L. (2009). *Hospitalizations Related to Childbirth, 2006* (Statistical Brief 71). Healthcare Cost and Utilization Project.
https://pubmed.ncbi.nlm.nih.gov/21510028/.
[7] The American College of Obstetricians and Gynecologists. (2010, August). *Practice Bulletin: Vaginal Birth After Previous Cesarean Delivery*. Maryland Department of Health. https://health.maryland.gov/midwives/Documents/ACOG%20VBAC.pdf.
[8] Hurst, A. (2021, May 3). *The Cost of a C-Section Is More Than $9,000 Greater on Average Than a Vaginal Delivery*. ValuePenguin.com.
https://www.valuepenguin.com/cost-of-vaginal-births-vs-c-sections.
[9] Swain, J. E., & Tasgin, E. (2008). Maternal brain response to own baby-cry is affected by cesarean section delivery. *Journal of Child Psychology and Psychiatry*, *49*(10), 1042-1052. https://doi.org/10.1111/j.1469-7610.2008.01963.x.
[10] *The World Factbook, 2023 Archive, Infant mortality rate*. (2024). CIA.gov.
https://www.cia.gov/the-world-factbook/about/archives/2023/field/infant-mortality-rate/country-comparison/.

[11] Johnson, K. C., & Daviss, B. (2005). Outcomes of planned home births with certified professional midwives: Large prospective study in North America. *BMJ*, *330*(7505), 1416. https://doi.org/10.1136/bmj.330.7505.1416.
[12] Cheyney, M., & Bovbjerg, M. (2014). Outcomes of care for 16,924 planned home births in the United States: The midwives alliance of North America statistics project, 2004 to 2009. *Journal of Midwifery & Women's Health*, *59*(1), 17-27. https://doi.org/10.1111/jmwh.12172.
[13] National Center for Health Statistics. (1998, May 19). *New Study Shows Lower Mortality Rates for Infants Delivered By Certified Nurse Midwives*. CDC.gov. https://www.cdc.gov/nchs/pressroom/98news/midwife.htm.
[14] Kluger, J. (2009, May 16). *Doctors versus midwives: The birth wars rage on*. TIME. https://time.com/archive/6933514/doctors-versus-midwives-the-birth-wars-rage-on/.
[15] Ibid.

Chapter 19

[1] Albin, R. J. (2010, March 9). The Great Prostate Mistake. *The New York Times*, Opinion.
https://www.nytimes.com/2010/03/10/opinion/10Ablin.html.
[2] Ablin, R. J., & Piana, R. (2014). *The great prostate hoax: How big medicine hijacked the PSA test and caused a public health disaster*. Macmillan.
[3] Mahar, M. (2010, March 10). *The doctor who invented PSA test calls it "a profit-driven public health disaster"*. HealthBeat Blog. https://www.healthbeatblog.com/2010/03/the-doctor-who-invented-psa-test-calls-it-a-profitdriven-public-health-disaster-why-this-is-good-new.
[4] Andriole, G. L., & Crawford, E. D. (2009). Mortality results from a randomized prostate-cancer screening trial. *New England Journal of Medicine*, *360*(13), 1310-1319. https://doi.org/10.1056/NEJMoa0810696
[5] Moyer, V. (2012). Screening for prostate cancer: U.S. Preventive Services Task Force recommendation statement. *Annals of Internal Medicine*, *157*(2), 120-134. https://doi.org/10.7326/0003-4819-157-2-201207170-00464.
[6] Thompson, D. (2015, May 18). *Prostate cancer testing drops off after controversial guidelines*. HealthDay: Information for Healthier Living.
https://www.healthday.com/health-news/general-health/prostate-cancer-testing-drops-off-after-controversial-guidelines-699497.html.
[7] Yetman, D. (2024). *How common is prostate cancer? Statistics, outlook, and more*. Healthline. https://www.healthline.com/health/prostate-cancer/how-common-is-prostate-cancer.
[8] Drach, G. W. (1975). Prostatitis: Man's hidden infection. *The Urologic Clinics of North America*, *2*(3), 499-520. https://pubmed.ncbi.nlm.nih.gov/52931/.
[9] Ibid.
[10] Nickel, J. C., & Downey, J. (1999). Repetitive prostatic massage therapy for chronic refractory prostatitis: the Philippine experience. *Techniques in Urology*, *5*(3), 146-151. https://pubmed.ncbi.nlm.nih.gov/10527258/.

[11] Rider, J. R., & Wilson, K. M. (2016). Ejaculation frequency and risk of prostate cancer: Updated results with an additional decade of follow-up. *European Urology*, *70*(6), 974-982. https://doi.org/10.1016/j.eururo.2016.03.027.
[12] Giles, G. G., & Severi, G. (2003). Sexual factors and prostate cancer. *BJU International*, *92*(3), 211-216. https://doi.org/10.1046/j.1464-410x.2003.04319.x.
[13] Sinnott, J. A., & Brumberg, K. (2018). Differential gene expression in prostate tissue according to ejaculation frequency. *European Urology*, *74*(5), 545-548. https://doi.org/10.1016/j.eururo.2018.05.006.

Chapter 20

[1] *Low testosterone*. (2024). Urology Care Foundation. https://www.urologyhealth.org/urology-a-z/l/low-testosterone.
[2] Layton, J. B., & Kim, Y. (2017). Association between direct-to-Consumer advertising and testosterone testing and initiation in the United States, 2009-2013. *JAMA*, *317*(11), 1159. https://doi.org/10.1001/jama.2016.21041.
[3] Travison, T. G., & Araujo, A. B. (2007). A population-level decline in serum testosterone levels in American men. *The Journal of Clinical Endocrinology & Metabolism*, *92*(1), 196-202. https://doi.org/10.1210/jc.2006-1375.
[4]·Nordal, E. (2010, May 12). *Testosterone levels decreasing in Danish men*. IceNews - Daily News | News in the Nordics. https://www.icenews.is/2010/05/17/testosterone-levels-decreasing-in-danish-men/#axzz4f1HF2xrr.
[5] Wang, S. (2013, July 15). The Decline in Male Fertility: Scientists puzzle over declining sperm counts; a 'crisis' or not enough data? *The Wall Street Journal*. https://www.wsj.com/articles/SB10001424127887323394504578607641775723354.
[6] Fain, E., & Weatherford, C. (2016). Comparative study of millennials' (age 20-34 years) grip and lateral pinch with the norms. *Journal of Hand Therapy*, *29*(4), 483-488. https://doi.org/10.1016/j.jht.2015.12.006.
[7] Leong, D. P., & Teo, K. K. (2015). Prognostic value of grip strength: Findings from the prospective urban rural epidemiology (PURE) study. *The Lancet*, *386*(9990), 266-273. https://doi.org/10.1016/s0140-6736(14)62000-6.
[8] Adams, N. R. (1995). Detection of the effects of phytoestrogens on sheep and cattle. *Journal of Animal Science*, *73*(5), 1509-1515. https://doi.org/10.2527/1995.7351509x.
[9] Chapin, R. (1996). Endocrine modulation of reproduction. *Fundamental and Applied Toxicology*, *29*(1), 1-17. https://doi.org/10.1006/faat.1996.0001.
[10] L'Office Federal de la Sante Publique, (1992). *Bulletin de l'office federal de la sante publique*. No. 28.
[11] Chavarro, J. E., & Toth, T. L. (2008). Soy food and isoflavone intake in relation to semen quality parameters among men from an infertility clinic. *Human Reproduction*, *23*(11), 2584-2590. https://doi.org/10.1093/humrep/den243.
[12] Smith, J. (2011, May 25). *Genetically modified soy linked to sterility, infant mortality in hamsters*. HuffPost. https://www.huffpost.com/entry/genetically-modified-soy_b_544575.
[13] Shahbandeh, M. (2022, December 16). *U.S. genetically modified crops: Percentage of total acreage 2020*. Statista. https://www.statista.com/statistics/217108/level-of-genetically-modified-crops-in-the-us/.

---

[14] La Vignera, S., & Condorelli, R. A. (2012). Effects of the exposure to mobile phones on male reproduction: A review of the literature. *Journal of Andrology*, *33*(3), 350-356. https://doi.org/10.2164/jandrol.111.014373.

[15] Davoudi, M. (2002). The influence of electromagnetic waves on sperm motility. *Journal fur Urologie und Urogynakologie*, 9(3), 18-22. https://www.researchgate.net/publication/285841428_The_influence_of_electromagnetic_waves.

[16] Agarwal, A., & Deepinder, F. (2008). Effect of cell phone usage on semen analysis in men attending infertility clinic: An observational study. *Fertility and Sterility*, *89*(1), 124-128. https://doi.org/10.1016/j.fertnstert.2007.01.166.

[17] *EWG's guide to safer cell phone use*. (2013, August 27). Environmental Working Group. https://www.ewg.org/research/ewgs-guide-safer-cell-phone-use.

[18] Lardinois, C. K., & Mazzaferri, E. L. (1985). Cimetidine blocks testosterone synthesis. *Archives of Internal Medicine*, *145*(5), 920-922. https://doi.org/10.1001/archinte.145.5.920.

[19] Pont, A. (1982). Ketoconazole blocks testosterone synthesis. *Archives of Internal Medicine*, *142*(12), 2137-2140. https://doi.org/10.1001/archinte.142.12.2137.

[20] Schooling, C. M., & Au Yeung, S. L. (2013). The effect of statins on testosterone in men and women, a systematic review and meta-analysis of randomized controlled trials. *BMC Medicine*, *11*(1). https://doi.org/10.1186/1741-7015-11-57.

[21] Cone, E. J., & Johnson, R. E. (1986). Acute effects of smoking marijuana on hormones, subjective effects and performance in male human subjects. *Pharmacology Biochemistry and Behavior*, *24*(6), 1749-1754. https://doi.org/10.1016/0091-3057(86)90515-0.

[22] *European Journal of Pharmacology*, (1974), 26:111-114; Endokrinologie, (1977), 69:299-305 https://www.sciencedirect.com/journal/european-journal-of-pharmacology/vol/26/issue/1.

[23] Gettler, L. T., & McDade, T. W. (2011). Longitudinal evidence that fatherhood decreases testosterone in human males. *Proceedings of the National Academy of Sciences*, *108*(39), 16194-16199. https://doi.org/10.1073/pnas.1105403108.

[24] Nierengarten, M. B. (2019, June 12). *Fathers' influence on development and well-being of children*. Contemporary Pediatrics. https://www.contemporarypediatrics.com/view/fathers-influence-development-and-well-being-children.

[25] Teicholz, N. (2022). A short history of saturated fat: The making and unmaking of a scientific consensus. *Current Opinion in Endocrinology, Diabetes & Obesity*, *30*(1), 65-71. https://doi.org/10.1097/med.0000000000000791.

[26] Ibid.

[27] McVoy, M. (2011, April 11). *Cholesterol: Your body is incapable of making hormones without it*. Metabolic Healing. https://metabolichealing.com/cholesterol-your-body-is-incapable-of-making-hormones-without-it.

[28] Wang, C., & Catlin, D. H. (2005). Low-fat high-fiber diet decreased serum and urine androgens in men. *The Journal of Clinical Endocrinology & Metabolism*, *90*(6), 3550-3559. https://doi.org/10.1210/jc.2004-1530.

[29] Hämäläinen, E., & Adlercreutz, H. (1984). Diet and serum sex hormones in healthy men. *Journal of Steroid Biochemistry*, *20*(1), 459-464. https://doi.org/10.1016/0022-4731(84)90254-1.

[30] Schreurs, B. G. (2010). The effects of cholesterol on learning and memory. *Neuroscience & Biobehavioral Reviews*, *34*(8), 1366-1379. https://doi.org/10.1016/j.neubiorev.2010.04.010.
[31] Mielke, M. M., & Zandi, P. P. (2005). High total cholesterol levels in late life associated with a reduced risk of dementia. *Neurology*, *64*(10), 1689-1695. https://doi.org/10.1212/01.wnl.0000161870.78572.a5.
[32] ZELIGS, M. A. (2009). Diet and estrogen status: The cruciferous connection. *Journal of Medicinal Food*, *1*(2), 67-82. https://doi.org/10.1089/jmf.1998.1.67.
[33] Kijima, I., & Phung, S. (2006). Grape seed extract is an Aromatase inhibitor and a suppressor of Aromatase expression. *Cancer Research*, *66*(11), 5960-5967. https://doi.org/10.1158/0008-5472.can-06-0053.
[34] Caronia, L. M., & Dwyer, A. A. (2013). Abrupt decrease in serum testosterone levels after an oral glucose load in men: Implications for screening for hypogonadism. *Clinical Endocrinology*, *78*(2), 291-296. https://doi.org/10.1111/j.1365-2265.2012.04486.x.
[35] Kraemer, W., & Gordon, S. (1991). Endogenous anabolic hormonal and growth factor responses to heavy resistance exercise in males and females. *International Journal of Sports Medicine*, *12*(2), 228-235. https://doi.org/10.1055/s-2007-1024673.
[36] Ibid.
[37] Hackney, A. C., & Hosick, K. P. (2012). Testosterone responses to intensive interval versus steady-state endurance exercise. *Journal of Endocrinological Investigation*, *35*(11), 947-950. https://doi.org/10.1007/bf03346740.
[38] Stokes, K., & Nevill, M. (2002). The time course of the human growth hormone response to a 6 S and a 30 S cycle ergometer sprint. *Journal of Sports Sciences*, *20*(6), 487-494. https://doi.org/10.1080/02640410252925152.
[39] Godfrey, R. J., & Madgwick, Z. (2003). The exercise-induced growth hormone response in athletes. *Sports Medicine*, *33*(8), 599-613. https://doi.org/10.2165/00007256-200333080-00005.
[40] Carney, D. R., & Cuddy, A. J. (2010). Power posing: brief nonverbal displays affect neuroendocrine levels and risk tolerance. *Psychological Science*, *21*(10), 1363-1368. https://doi.org/10.1177/0956797610383437.
[41] Jobling, S., & Reynolds, T. (1995). A variety of environmentally persistent chemicals, including some phthalate plasticizers, are weakly Estrogenic. *Environmental Health Perspectives*, *103*(6), 582. https://doi.org/10.2307/3432434.
[42] Routledge, E. J., & Parker, J. (1998). Some alkyl hydroxy benzoate preservatives (Parabens) are Estrogenic. *Toxicology and Applied Pharmacology*, *153*(1), 12-19. https://doi.org/10.1006/taap.1998.8544.
[43] Prasad, A. S., & Mantzoros, C. S. (1996). Zinc status and serum testosterone levels of healthy adults. *Nutrition*, *12*(5), 344-348. https://doi.org/10.1016/s0899-9007(96)80058-x.
[44] Netter, A., & Nahoul, K. (1981). Effect of zinc administration on plasma testosterone, Dihydrotestosterone, and sperm count. *Archives of Andrology*, *7*(1), 69-73. https://doi.org/10.3109/01485018109009378.
[45] Kilic, M., & Baltaci, A. K. (2006). The effect of exhaustion exercise on thyroid hormones and testosterone levels of elite athletes receiving oral zinc. *Neuro Endocrinology Letters*, *27*(1-2), 247-252. https://pubmed.ncbi.nlm.nih.gov/16648789/.

[46] Wehr, E., & Pilz, S. (2010). Association of vitamin D status with serum androgen levels in men. *Clinical Endocrinology*, *73*(2), 243-248. https://doi.org/10.1111/j.1365-2265.2009.03777.x.
[47] Pilz, S., & Frisch, S. (2010). Effect of vitamin D supplementation on testosterone levels in men. *Hormone and Metabolic Research*, *43*(03), 223-225. https://doi.org/10.1055/s-0030-1269854.
[48] Topo, E., & Soricelli, A. (2009). The role and molecular mechanism of D-aspartic acid in the release and synthesis of LH and testosterone in humans and rats. *Reproductive Biology and Endocrinology*, *7*(1), 120. https://doi.org/10.1186/1477-7827-7-120.
[49] D'Aniello, G., Ronsini, S., Notari, T., Grieco, N., Infante, V., D'Angel, N., Mascia, F., Fiore, M. M., Fisher, G., & D'Aniello, A. (2012). D-aspartate, a key element for the improvement of sperm quality. *Advances in Sexual Medicine*, *2*(1), 47-53. https://doi.org/10.4236/asm.2012.24008.
[50] Sellandi, T., & Thakar, A. (2012). Clinical study of Tribulus terrestris Linn. in Oligozoospermia: A double blind study. *AYU (An international quarterly journal of research in Ayurveda)*, *33*(3), 356. https://doi.org/10.4103/0974-8520.108822.
[51] Rogerson, S., & Riches, C. J. (2007). The effect of five weeks of Tribulus terrestris supplementation on muscle strength and body composition during Preseason training in elite Rugby league players. *The Journal of Strength and Conditioning Research*, *21*(2), 348. https://doi.org/10.1519/r-18395.1.
[52] Wilborn, C., & Taylor, L. (2010). Effects of a purported Aromatase and 5 α-reductase inhibitor on hormone profiles in college-age men. *International Journal of Sport Nutrition and Exercise Metabolism*, *20*(6), 457-465. https://doi.org/10.1123/ijsnem.20.6.457.
[53] Steels, E., & Rao, A. (2011). Physiological aspects of male libido enhanced by standardized *Trigonella foenum-graecum* extract and mineral formulation. *Phytotherapy Research*, *25*(9), 1294-1300. https://doi.org/10.1002/ptr.3360.
[54] Ghlissi, Z., & Atheymen, R. (2013). Antioxidant and androgenic effects of dietary ginger on reproductive function of male diabetic rats. *International Journal of Food Sciences and Nutrition*, *64*(8), 974-978. https://doi.org/10.3109/09637486.2013.812618.
[55] Khaki, A. A., & Fathiazad, F. (2009). The effects of ginger on spermatogenesis and sperm parameters of rat. *International Journal of Reproductive Medicine*, *7*(1), 7-12. https://www.bioline.org.br/abstract?rm09002.
[56] Maris, W. A., & Najam, W. S. (2012). The effect of ginger on semen parameters and serum FSH, LH & testosterone of infertile men. *The Medical Journal of Tikrit University*, *18*(182). https://www.iasj.net/iasj?func=fulltext&aId=71548.
[57] Martina, V., & Benso, A. (2006). Short-term dehydroepiandrosterone treatment increases platelet cGMP production in elderly male subjects. *Clinical Endocrinology*, *64*(3), 260-264. https://doi.org/10.1111/j.1365-2265.2006.02454.x.
[58] Morales, A., & Black, A. (2009). Androgens and sexual function: A placebo-controlled, randomized, double-blind study of testosterone*vs.* dehydroepiandrosterone in men with sexual dysfunction and androgen deficiency. *The Aging Male*, *12*(4), 104-112. https://doi.org/10.3109/13685530903294388.
[59] Mahdi, A. A., & Shukla, K. K. (2011). Withania somnifera improves semen quality in stress-related male fertility. *Evidence-Based Complementary and Alternative Medicine*, *29*(12), 341-349. https://doi.org/10.1093/ecam/nep138.

[60] Wankhede, S., & Langade, D. (2015). Examining the effect of Withania somnifera supplementation on muscle strength and recovery: a randomized controlled trial. *Journal of the International Society of Sports Nutrition*, *12*(1), 43. https://doi.org/10.1186/s12970-015-0104-9
[61] Zhang, Y., & Cao, H. (2013). Curcumin inhibits endometriosis endometrial cells by reducing estradiol production. *Iranian Journal of Reproductive Medicine*, *11*(5), 415-422. https://pubmed.ncbi.nlm.nih.gov/24639774/.
[62] Soni, K. B., & Kuttan, R. (1992). Effect of oral curcumin administration on serum peroxides and cholesterol levels in human volunteers. *Indian Journal of Physiology and Pharmacology*, *36*(4), 273-275. https://pubmed.ncbi.nlm.nih.gov/1291482/.
[63] Bartik, L., & Whitfield, G. K. (2010). Curcumin: A novel nutritionally derived ligand of the vitamin D receptor with implications for colon cancer chemoprevention. *The Journal of Nutritional Biochemistry*, *21*(12), 1153-1161. https://doi.org/10.1016/j.jnutbio.2009.09.012.
[64] Di Pierro, F., & Bressan, A. (2015). Potential role of bioavailable curcumin in weight loss and omental adipose tissue decrease: preliminary data of a randomized, controlled trial in overweight people with metabolic syndrome. Preliminary study. *European Review for Medical and Pharmacological Sciences*, *19*(21), 2195-2202. https://pubmed.ncbi.nlm.nih.gov/26592847/.
[65] Kuptniratsaikul, V., & Dajpratham, P. (2014). Efficacy and safety of curcuma domestica extracts compared with ibuprofen in patients with knee osteoarthritis: A multicenter study. *Clinical Interventions in Aging*, *20*(9), 451-458. https://doi.org/10.2147/cia.s58535.
[66] Ghorbani, Z., & Hekmatdoost, A. (2014). Anti-hyperglycemic and insulin sensitizer effects of turmeric and its principle constituent curcumin. *International Journal of Endocrinology and Metabolism*, *12*(4), e18081. https://doi.org/10.5812/ijem.18081.
[67] Shoba, G., & Joy, D. (1998). Influence of piperine on the pharmacokinetics of curcumin in animals and human volunteers. *Planta Medica*, *64*(4), 353-356. https://doi.org/10.1055/s-2006-957450.
[68] Yang, J., & Wu, G. (2010). Effects of taurine on male reproduction in rats of different ages. *Journal of Biomedical Science*, 17 Suppl 1(Suppl 1):S9. https://doi.org/10.1186/1423-0127-17-s1-s9.
[69] Yang, J., & Wu, G. (2010). CSD mRNA expression in rat testis and the effect of taurine on testosterone secretion. *Amino Acids*, *39*(1), 155-160. https://doi.org/10.1007/s00726-009-0388-7.

Chapter 21

[1] Trevathan, W. R., & Burleson, M. H. (1993). No evidence for menstrual synchrony in lesbian couples. *Psychoneuroendocrinology*, *18*(5-6), 425-435. https://doi.org/10.1016/0306-4530(93)90017-f.
[2] Stern, K., & McClintock, M. K. (1998). Regulation of ovulation by human pheromones. *Nature*, *392*(6672), 177-179. https://doi.org/10.1038/32408.
[3] Benziger, D. P., & Edelson, J. (1983). Absorption from the vagina. *Drug Metabolism Reviews*, *14*(2), 137-168. https://doi.org/10.3109/03602538308991387.

[4] Gallup, G. G., & Burch, R. L. (2002). Does semen have antidepressant properties? *Archives of Sexual Behavior*, *31*(3), 289-293. https://doi.org/10.1023/a:1015257004839.
[5] Ibid.
[6] Valsa, J., & Skandhan, K. P. (1992). Cholesterol in normal and pathological seminal plasma. *Panminerva Medica*, *34*(4), 160-162. https://pubmed.ncbi.nlm.nih.gov/1293543/.
[7] Brotherton, J. (1990). Cortisol and transcortin in human seminal plasma and amniotic fluid as estimated by modern specific assays. *Andrologia*, *22*(3), 197-204. https://doi.org/10.1111/j.1439-0272.1990.tb01966.x.
[8] Nelson, R. J., & Kriegsfeld, L. J. (2022). *An introduction to behavioral endocrinology* (5th ed.). Sinauer Associates.
[9] Ney, P. (1986). The intravaginal absorption of male generated hormones and their possible effect on female behaviour. *Medical Hypotheses*, *20*(2), 221-231. https://doi.org/10.1016/0306-9877(86)90128-3.
[10] Asch, R. H., & Fernandez, E. O. (1984). Peptide and steroid hormone concentrations in human seminal plasma. *International Journal of Fertility*, *29*(1), 25-32. https://pubmed.ncbi.nlm.nih.gov/6146580/.
[11] Wester, R. C., & Noonan, P. K. (1980). Variations in percutaneous absorption of testosterone in the rhesus monkey due to anatomic site of application and frequency of application. *Archives of Dermatological Research*, *267*(3), 229-235. https://doi.org/10.1007/bf00403844.
[12] Morris, N. M., & Udry, J. R. (1987). Marital sex frequency and midcycle female testosterone. *Archives of Sexual Behavior*, *16*(1), 27-37. https://doi.org/10.1007/bf01541839.
[13] Gallup, G. G., & Burch, R. L. (2002). Does semen have antidepressant properties? *Archives of Sexual Behavior*, *31*(3), 289-293. https://doi.org/10.1023/a:1015257004839.
[14] Ney, P. (1986). The intravaginal absorption of male generated hormones and their possible effect on female behaviour. *Medical Hypotheses*, *20*(2), 221-231. https://doi.org/10.1016/0306-9877(86)90128-3.
[15] Luboshitzky, R., & Shen-Orr, Z. (2002). Seminal plasma melatonin and gonadal steroids concentrations in normal men. *Archives of Andrology*, *48*(3), 225-232. https://doi.org/10.1080/01485010252869324.
[16] Schiff, I., & Tulchinsky, D. (1977). Vaginal absorption of Estrone and 17β-Estradiol. *Fertility and Sterility*, *28*(10), 1063-1066. https://doi.org/10.1016/s0015-0282(16)42855-4.
[17] Rigg, L. A., & Milanes, B. (1977). Efficacy of Intravaginal and intranasal administration of Micronized estradiol-17β1. *The Journal of Clinical Endocrinology & Metabolism*, *45*(6), 1261-1264. https://doi.org/10.1210/jcem-45-6-1261.
[18] Nelson, R. J., & Kriegsfeld, L. J. (2022). *An introduction to behavioral endocrinology* (5th ed.). Sinauer Associates.
[19] Burch, R. L., & Gallup, G. G. (2006). Chapter 8 - The psychobiology of human semen. *Female Infidelity and Paternal Uncertainty*, 141-172. https://doi.org/10.1017/cbo9780511617812.008.
[20] Sherwin, B. (1985). Sex steroids and affect in the surgical menopause: A double-blind, cross-over study. *Psychoneuroendocrinology*, *10*(3), 325-335. https://doi.org/10.1016/0306-4530(85)90009-5.

---

[21] Schneider, L. S., & Small, G. W. (1997). Estrogen replacement and response to fluoxetine in a multicenter geriatric depression trial. *American Journal of Geriatric Psychiatry*, *5*(2), 97-106. https://doi.org/10.1097/00019442-199721520-00002.

[22] Lebowitz, B. D. (1997). Estrogen in geriatric psychopharmacology. *Psychopharmacology Bulletin*, *33*(2), 287-288. https://pubmed.ncbi.nlm.nih.gov/9230644/.

[23] Coope, J., & Thomson, J. M. (1975). Effects of "natural oestrogen" replacement therapy on menopausal symptoms and blood clotting. *BMJ*, *4*(5989), 139-143. https://doi.org/10.1136/bmj.4.5989.139.

[24] Golub, S. (1976). The magnitude of premenstrual anxiety and depression. *Psychosomatic Medicine*, *38*(1), 4-12. https://doi.org/10.1097/00006842-197601000-00002.

[25] Bancroft, J., & Sanders, D. (1983). Mood, sexuality, hormones, and the menstrual cycle. III. Sexuality and the role of androgens. *Psychosomatic Medicine*, *45*(6), 509-516. https://doi.org/10.1097/00006842-198312000-00005.

[26] Lawrie, T. A., & Herxheimer, A. (2000). Oestrogens and progestogens for preventing and treating postnatal depression. *The Cochrane Database of Systematic Reviews*, *2*(001690). https://doi.org/10.1002/14651858.CD001690.

[27] Ney, P. (1986). The intravaginal absorption of male generated hormones and their possible effect on female behaviour. *Medical Hypotheses*, *20*(2), 221-231. https://doi.org/10.1016/0306-9877(86)90128-3.

[28] Sheth, A. R., & Shah, G. V. (1976). Levels of luteinizing hormone in semen of Fertile and infertile men and possible significance of luteinizing hormone in sperm metabolism. *Fertility and Sterility*, *27*(8), 933-936. https://doi.org/10.1016/s0015-0282(16)42015-7.

[29] Asch, R. H., & Fernandez, E. O. (1984). Peptide and steroid hormone concentrations in human seminal plasma. *International Journal of Fertility*, *29*(1), 25-32. https://pubmed.ncbi.nlm.nih.gov/6146580/.

[30] Nelson, R. J., & Kriegsfeld, L. J. (2022). *An introduction to behavioral endocrinology* (5th ed.). Sinauer Associates.

[31] Keller, P., & Riedmann, R. (1981). Oestrogens, gonadotropins and prolactin after intra-vaginal administration of oestriol in post-menopausal women. *Maturitas*, *3*(1), 47-53. https://doi.org/10.1016/0378-5122(81)90019-0.

[32] Grattan, D. R. (2001). Chapter 11 the actions of prolactin in the brain during pregnancy and lactation. *Progress in Brain Research*, 153-171. https://doi.org/10.1016/s0079-6123(01)33012-1.

[33] Golden, R. (2002). A longitudinal study of Serotonergic function in depression. *Neuropsychopharmacology*, *26*(5), 653-659. https://doi.org/10.1016/s0893-133x(01)00406-7.

[34] Hendrick, V., & Altshuler, L. L. (1998). Hormonal changes in the postpartum and implications for postpartum depression. *Psychosomatics*, *39*(2), 93-101. https://doi.org/10.1016/s0033-3182(98)71355-6.

[35] Derzko, C. M. (1990). Role of danazol in relieving the premenstrual syndrome. *The Journal of Reproductive Medicine*, *35*(1Supp), 97-102. https://pubmed.ncbi.nlm.nih.gov/2404119/.

[36] Sandberg, F., & Ingelman-Sundberg, A. (1968). The absorption of tritium-labelled prostaglandin E₁ from the vagina of non-pregnant women. *Acta Obstetricia et Gynecologica Scandinavica, 47*(1), 22-26. https://doi.org/10.3109/00016346809157462.
[37] Kelly, R. (1995). Contraception: Immunosuppressive mechanisms in semen: implications for contraception. *Human Reproduction, 10*(7), 1686-1693. https://doi.org/10.1093/oxfordjournals.humrep.a136156.
[38] Maegawa, M., & Kamada, M. (2002). A repertoire of cytokines in human seminal plasma. *Journal of Reproductive Immunology, 54*(1-2), 33-42. https://doi.org/10.1016/s0165-0378(01)00063-8.
[39] Zalata, A., & Hafez, T. (1995). Evaluation of β-endorphin and interleukin-6 in seminal plasma of patients with certain andrological diseases. *Human Reproduction, 10*(12), 3161-3165. https://doi.org/10.1093/oxfordjournals.humrep.a135879.
[40] Mungan, N. A., & Mungan, G. (2001). Effect of seminal plasma calcitonin levels on sperm motility. *Archives of Andrology, 47*(2), 113-117. https://doi.org/10.1080/014850101316901316
[41] Stahl, S. M. (2013). *Stahl's essential psychopharmacology: Neuroscientific basis and practical applications.* Cambridge University Press.
[42] Turner, R. A., & Altemus, M. (1999). Preliminary research on plasma oxytocin in normal cycling women: Investigating emotion and interpersonal distress. *Psychiatry, 62*(2), 97-113. https://doi.org/10.1080/00332747.1999.11024859.
[43] Nelson, R. J., & Kriegsfeld, L. J. (2022). *An introduction to behavioral endocrinology* (5th ed.). Sinauer Associates.
[44] Winslow, J. T., & Hastings, N. (1993). A role for central vasopressin in pair bonding in monogamous prairie voles. *Nature, 365*(6446), 545-548. https://doi.org/10.1038/365545a0.
[45] De Medeiros, S. F., & Amato, F. (1992). Distribution of the β-core human chorionic gonadotrophin fragment in human body fluids. *Journal of Endocrinology, 135*(1), 175-188. https://doi.org/10.1677/joe.0.1350175.
[46] Seppala, M., & Koskimies, A. I. (1985). Pregnancy proteins in seminal plasma, seminal vesicles, Preovulatory follicular fluid, and Ovary. *Annals of the New York Academy of Sciences, 442*(1), 212-226. https://doi.org/10.1111/j.1749-6632.1985.tb37522.x.
[47] Brotherton, J. (2009). Ferritin: Another pregnancy-specific protein in human seminal plasma and amniotic fluid, as estimated by six methods: Ferritin: ein weiteres schwangerschaftsspezifisches Eiweiß in menschlichem Seminalplasma und Fruchtwasser. *Andrologia, 22*(6), 597-607. https://doi.org/10.1111/j.1439-0272.1990.tb02062.x.
[48] De Medeiros, S. F., & Amato, F. (1992). Distribution of the β-core human chorionic gonadotrophin fragment in human body fluids. *Journal of Endocrinology, 135*(1), 175-188. https://doi.org/10.1677/joe.0.1350175.
[49] MacLennan, A. H. (1991). The role of the hormone relaxin in human reproduction and pelvic girdle relaxation. *Scandinavian Journal of Rheumatology Supplement, 88*, 7-15. https://pubmed.ncbi.nlm.nih.gov/2011710/.
[50] Stewart, D. R., & Celniker, A. C. (1990). Relaxin in the Peri-implantation period. *The Journal of Clinical Endocrinology & Metabolism, 70*(6), 1771-1773. https://doi.org/10.1210/jcem-70-6-1771.

[51] MacLennan, A. H. (1991). The role of the hormone relaxin in human reproduction and pelvic girdle relaxation. *Scandinavian Journal of Rheumatology Supplement*, *88*, 7-15. https://pubmed.ncbi.nlm.nih.gov/2011710.
[52] Burch, R. L., & Gallup, G. G. (2006). Chapter 8 - The psychobiology of human semen. *Female Infidelity and Paternal Uncertainty*, 141-172. https://doi.org/10.1017/cbo9780511617812.008.
[53] Pekary, A. E., & Hershman, J. M. (1983). Human semen contains thyrotropin releasing hormone (TRH), a TRH-homologous peptide, and TRH-binding substances. *Journal of Andrology*, *4*(6), 399-407. https://doi.org/10.1002/j.1939-4640.1983.tb00767.x.
[54] Gkonos, P. J., & Kwok, C. K. (1994). Identification of the human seminal TRH-like peptide pglu-phe-Pro-NH2 in normal human prostate. *Peptides*, *15*(7), 1281-1283. https://doi.org/10.1016/0196-9781(94)90154-6.
[55] Roy-Byrne, P., & Rubinow, D. R. (1984). Possible antidepressant effect of oral contraceptives: case report. *The Journal of Clinical Psychiatry*, *45*(8), 350-352. https://pubmed.ncbi.nlm.nih.gov/6540262/.
[56] Stahl, S. M. (2013). *Stahl's essential psychopharmacology: Neuroscientific basis and practical applications*. Cambridge University Press.
[57] Gonzales, G. F., & Garcia-Hjarles, M. A. (1989). Blood serotonin levels and male infertility. *Archives of Andrology*, *22*(1), 85-89. https://doi.org/10.3109/01485018908986755.
[58] Weaver, D. R. (1997). Reproductive safety of melatonin: A "Wonder drug" to wonder about. *Journal of Biological Rhythms*, *12*(6), 682-689. https://doi.org/10.1177/074873049701200625.
[59] Burch, R. L., & Gallup, G. G. (2006). Chapter 8 - The psychobiology of human semen. *Female Infidelity and Paternal Uncertainty*, 141-172. https://doi.org/10.1017/cbo9780511617812.008.
[60] Souêtre, E. (1987). Seasonality of suicides: Environmental, sociological and biological covariations. *Journal of Affective Disorders*, *13*(3), 215-225. https://doi.org/10.1016/0165-0327(87)90040-1.
[61] Lewy, A., & Wehr, T. (1981). Manic-depressive patients may be supersensitive to light. *The Lancet*, *317*(8216), 383-384. https://doi.org/10.1016/s0140-6736(81)91697-4.
[62] Fait, G., & Vered, Y. (2001). High levels of catecholamines in human semen: A preliminary study. *Andrologia*, *33*(6), 347-350. https://doi.org/10.1046/j.1439-0272.2001.00461.x.
[63] Stahl, S. M. (2013). *Stahl's essential psychopharmacology: Neuroscientific basis and practical applications*. Cambridge University Press.
[64] Burleson, M. H., & Gregory, W. (1991). Heterosexual activity and cycle length variability: Effect of gynecological maturity. *Physiology & Behavior*, *50*(4), 863-866. https://doi.org/10.1016/0031-9384(91)90032-j.
[65] Creinin, M. D. (2000). Medical abortion regimens: Historical context and overview. *American Journal of Obstetrics and Gynecology*, *183*(2), S3-S9. https://doi.org/10.1067/mob.2000.107948.
[66] Marashi, V., & Rülicke, T. (2012). The Bruce effect in Norway Rats. *Biology of Reproduction*, *86*(1). https://doi.org/10.1095/biolreprod.111.093104.
[67] Nelson, R. J., & Kriegsfeld, L. J. (2022). *An introduction to behavioral endocrinology* (5th ed.). Sinauer Associates.

[68] Argyriou, A., & Prast, H. (1998). Melatonin facilitates short-term memory. *European Journal of Pharmacology*, *349*(2-3), 159-162. https://doi.org/10.1016/s0014-2999(98)00300-8.
[69] Burch, R. L., & Gallup, G. G. (2006). Chapter 8 - The psychobiology of human semen. *Female Infidelity and Paternal Uncertainty*, 141-172. https://doi.org/10.1017/cbo9780511617812.008.

Chapter 22

[1] Power to Decide. (2016). *Parent Power, Survey Says*. PowertoDecide.org. https://powertodecide.org/what-we-do/information/resource-library/parent-power-october-2016-survey-says.
[2] Grossman, J. M., & Richer, A. M. (2018). Youth perspectives on sexuality communication with parents and extended family. *Family Relations*, *67*(3), 368-380. https://doi.org/10.1111/fare.12313.
[3] GuardChild. (2020). *Internet Statistics*. GuardChild.com. https://www.guardchild.com/statistics/.

Chapter 23

[1] Wolak, J., & Mitchell, K. (2007). Unwanted and wanted exposure to online pornography in a national sample of youth internet users. *Pediatrics*, *119*(2), 247-257. https://doi.org/10.1542/peds.2006-1891.
[2] Ibid.
[3] Kraus, S. W., & Russell, B. (2008). Early sexual experiences: The role of internet access and sexually explicit material. *CyberPsychology & Behavior*, *11*(2), 162-168. https://doi.org/10.1089/cpb.2007.0054.
[4] Wolak, J et al. (2007). Unwanted and wanted exposure to online pornography in a national sample of youth internet users. *Pediatrics*, 119(2), 247-257, doi: 10.1542/peds.2006-1891.
[5] Sabina, C., & Wolak, J. (2008). The nature and dynamics of internet pornography exposure for youth. *CyberPsychology & Behavior*, *11*(6), 691-693. https://doi.org/10.1089/cpb.2007.0179.
[6] Sun, C., & Bridges, A. (2014). Pornography and the male sexual script: An analysis of consumption and sexual relations. *Archives of Sexual Behavior*, *45*(4), 983-994. https://doi.org/10.1007/s10508-014-0391-2.
[7] Voon, V., & Mole, T. B. (2014). Neural correlates of sexual cue reactivity in individuals with and without compulsive sexual behaviours. *PLoS ONE*, *9*(7), e102419. https://doi.org/10.1371/journal.pone.0102419.
[8] Häggström-Nordin, E., & Sandberg, J. (2006). 'It's everywhere!' Young Swedish people's thoughts and reflections about pornography. *Scandinavian Journal of Caring Sciences*, *20*(4), 386-393. https://doi.org/10.1111/j.1471-6712.2006.00417.x.

[9] Alexy, E. M., & Burgess, A. W. (2009). Pornography use as a risk marker for an aggressive pattern of behavior among sexually reactive children and adolescents. *Journal of the American Psychiatric Nurses Association*, *14*(6), 442-453. https://doi.org/10.1177/1078390308327137.
[10] Schrimshaw, E. W., & Antebi-Gruszka, N. (2016). Viewing of internet-based sexually explicit media as a risk factor for Condomless anal sex among men who have sex with men in four U.S. cities. *PLOS ONE*, *11*(4), e0154439. https://doi.org/10.1371/journal.pone.0154439.
[11] Martellozzo, E., & Monaghan, A. (2016, June). *"I wasn't sure it was normal to watch it." A quantitative and qualitative examination of the mpact of online pornography on the values, attitudes, beliefs and behaviours of children and young people.* dera.ioe.acuk. https://dera.ioe.ac.uk/27973/1/MDX NSPCC OCC pornography report June 2016.pdf.
[12] Braun-Courville, D. K., & Rojas, M. (2009). Exposure to sexually explicit web sites and adolescent sexual attitudes and behaviors. *Journal of Adolescent Health*, *45*(2), 156-162. https://doi.org/10.1016/j.jadohealth.2008.12.004.
[13] Ibid.
[14] Coker, A. L., & Richter, D. L. (1994). Correlates and consequences of early initiation of sexual intercourse. *Journal of School Health*, *64*(9), 372-377. https://doi.org/10.1111/j.1746-1561.1994.tb06208.x.
[15] Kaestle, C. E. (2005). Young age at first sexual intercourse and sexually transmitted infections in adolescents and young adults. *American Journal of Epidemiology*, *161*(8), 774-780. https://doi.org/10.1093/aje/kwi095.
[16] Coker, A. L., & Richter, D. L. (1994). Correlates and consequences of early initiation of sexual intercourse. *Journal of School Health*, *64*(9), 372-377. https://doi.org/10.1111/j.1746-1561.1994.tb06208.x.
[17] Kail, R. V., & Cavanaugh, J. C. (2019). *Human development: A life-span view* (8th ed.). Cengage, Boston, MA.
[18] Morgan, E. M. (2011). Associations between young adults' use of sexually explicit materials and their sexual preferences, behaviors, and satisfaction. *Journal of Sex Research*, *48*(6), 520-530. https://doi.org/10.1080/00224499.2010.543960.
[19] Heywood, W., & Patrick, K. (2014). Associations between early first sexual intercourse and later sexual and reproductive outcomes: A systematic review of population-based data. *Archives of Sexual Behavior*, *44*(3), 531-569. https://doi.org/10.1007/s10508-014-0374-3.
[20] Stanley, N., & Barter, C. (2016). Pornography, sexual coercion and abuse and sexting in young people's intimate relationships: A European study. *Journal of Interpersonal Violence*, *33*(19), 2919-2944. https://doi.org/10.1177/0886260516633204.
[21] Peter, J., & Valkenburg, P. M. (2006). Adolescents' exposure to sexually explicit online material and recreational attitudes toward sex. *Journal of Communication*, *56*(4), 639-660. https://doi.org/10.1111/j.1460-2466.2006.00313.x.
[22] Heywood, W., & Patrick, K. (2014). Associations between early first sexual intercourse and later sexual and reproductive outcomes: A systematic review of population-based data. *Archives of Sexual Behavior*, *44*(3), 531-569. https://doi.org/10.1007/s10508-014-0374-3.
[23] Young, B. (2017, January 5). *The Impact of Timing of Pornography Exposure on Mental Health, Life Satisfaction, and Sexual Behavior*. BYU Scholars Archive. https://scholarsarchive.byu.edu/cgi/viewcontent.cgi?article=7727&context=etd.

[24] Wright, P. J., & Sun, C. (2017). Associative pathways between pornography consumption and reduced sexual satisfaction. *Sexual and Relationship Therapy, 34*(4), 422-439. https://doi.org/10.1080/14681994.2017.1323076.

[25] Shultz, D. (2016, August 26). *Divorce rates double when people start watching porn.* Science.com. https://www.science.org/content/article/divorce-rates-double-when-people-start-watching-porn.

[26] Daneback, K., & Træen, B. (2008). Use of pornography in a random sample of Norwegian heterosexual couples. *Archives of Sexual Behavior, 38*(5), 746-753. https://doi.org/10.1007/s10508-008-9314-4.

[27] Doran, K., & Price, J. (2014). Pornography and Marriage. *Journal of Family and Economic Issues, 35*, 489-498. https://doi.org/10.1007/s10834-014-9391-6.

[28] Lambert, N. M., & Negash, S. (2012). A love that doesn't last: Pornography consumption and weakened commitment to one's romantic partner. *Journal of Social and Clinical Psychology, 31*(4), 410-438. https://doi.org/10.1521/jscp.2012.31.4.410.

[29] Sun, C., & Bridges, A. (2014). Pornography and the male sexual script: An analysis of consumption and sexual relations. *Archives of Sexual Behavior, 45*(4), 983-994. https://doi.org/10.1007/s10508-014-0391-2.

[30] Wéry, A., & Billieux, J. (2016). Online sexual activities: An exploratory study of problematic and non-problematic usage patterns in a sample of men. *Computers in Human Behavior, 56*, 257-266. https://doi.org/10.1016/j.chb.2015.11.046.

[31] Lambert, N. M., & Negash, S. (2012). A love that doesn't last: Pornography consumption and weakened commitment to one's romantic partner. *Journal of Social and Clinical Psychology, 31*(4), 410-438. https://doi.org/10.1521/jscp.2012.31.4.410.

[32] Kaltiala-Heino, R., & Rimpel, M. (2001). Early puberty and early sexual activity are associated with bulimic-type eating pathology in middle adolescence11The full text of this article is available via JAH online at HTTP://www.elsevier.com/locate/ajpmonline. *Journal of Adolescent Health, 28*(4), 346-352. https://doi.org/10.1016/s1054-139x(01)00195-1.

[33] Sun, C., & Bridges, A. (2014). Pornography and the male sexual script: An analysis of consumption and sexual relations. *Archives of Sexual Behavior, 45*(4), 983-994. https://doi.org/10.1007/s10508-014-0391-2.

[34] Veale, D., & Miles, S. (2015). Am I normal? A systematic review and construction of nomograms for flaccid and erect penis length and circumference in up to 15 521 men. *BJU International, 115*(6), 978-986. https://doi.org/10.1111/bju.13010.

[35] Sun, C., & Bridges, A. (2014). Pornography and the male sexual script: An analysis of consumption and sexual relations. *Archives of Sexual Behavior, 45*(4), 983-994. https://doi.org/10.1007/s10508-014-0391-2.

[36] Perry, S. L., & Davis, J. T. (2017). Are pornography users more likely to experience a romantic breakup? Evidence from longitudinal data. *Sexuality & Culture, 21*(4), 1157-1176. https://doi.org/10.1007/s12119-017-9444-8.

[37] Stack, S., & Wasserman, I. (2004). Adult social bonds and use of internet pornography. *Social Science Quarterly, 85*(1), 75-88. https://doi.org/10.1111/j.0038-4941.2004.08501006.x.

Chapter 24

[1] Tacopino, J. (2016, May 19). *Not using transgender pronouns could get you fined.* New York Post. https://nypost.com/2016/05/19/city-issues-new-guidelines-on-transgender-pronouns.
[2] Singman, B. (2017, October 9). *New California law allows jail time for using wrong gender pronoun, sponsor denies that would happen.* Fox News. https://www.foxnews.com/politics/new-california-law-allows-jail-time-for-using-wrong-gender-pronoun-sponsor-denies-that-would-happen.
[3] Et al. (2017). An Issue Whose Time Has Come: Sex/Gender Influences on Nervous System Function. *Journal of Neuroscience Research, Jan./Feb. Spc1*, 1-791. https://onlinelibrary.wiley.com/toc/10974547/95/1-2.
[4] Prager, E. M. (2017). Addressing Sex as a Biological Variable. *Journal of Neuroscience Research*, *95*(1-2), 11. https://onlinelibrary.wiley.com/doi/10.1002/jnr.23979.
[5] Clayton, J. A. (2016, February 1). *Sex as a biological variable: A step toward stronger.* National Institutes of Health. https://orwh.od.nih.gov/about/director/messages/sex-biological-variable.
[6] Story, C. M. (2018, January 23). *Heart attack symptoms in men and women.* Healthline. https://www.healthline.com/health/heart-disease/heart-attack-symptoms.
[7] Todd, B. K., & Barry, J. A. (2016). Preferences for 'gender-typed' toys in boys and girls aged 9 to 32 Months. *Infant and Child Development*, *26*(3). https://doi.org/10.1002/icd.1986.
[8] Carter, D. B., & Levy, G. D. (1988). Cognitive aspects of early sex-role development: The influence of gender schemas on preschoolers' memories and preferences for sex-typed toys and activities. *Child Development*, *59*(3), 782. https://doi.org/10.2307/1130576.
[9] Berenbaum, S. A., & Hines, M. (1992). Early androgens are related to childhood sex-typed toy preferences. *Psychological Science*, *3*(3), 203-206. https://doi.org/10.1111/j.1467-9280.1992.tb00028.x.
[10] Williams, C. L., & Pleil, K. E. (2008). Toy story: Why do monkey and human males prefer trucks? Comment on "sex differences in rhesus monkey toy preferences parallel those of children.". *Hormones and Behavior*, *54*(3), 355-358. https://doi.org/10.1016/j.yhbeh.2008.05.003.
[11] Hassett, J. M., & Siebert, E. R. (2008). Sex differences in rhesus monkey toy preferences parallel those of children. *Hormones and Behavior*, *54*(3), 359-364. https://doi.org/10.1016/j.yhbeh.2008.03.008.
[12] Wheelock, M. D., & Hect, J. L. (2019). Sex differences in functional connectivity during fetal brain development. *Developmental Cognitive Neuroscience*, *36*(100632). https://doi.org/10.1016/j.dcn.2019.100632.
[13] Ruigrok, A. N., & Salimi-Khorshidi, G. (2014). A meta-analysis of sex differences in human brain structure. *Neuroscience & Biobehavioral Reviews*, *39*, 34-50. https://doi.org/10.1016/j.neubiorev.2013.12.004.
[14] Ingalhalikar, M., & Smith, A. (2013). Sex differences in the structural connectome of the human brain. *Proceedings of the National Academy of Sciences*, *111*(2), 823-828. https://doi.org/10.1073/pnas.1316909110.

[15] Anderson, N. E., & Harenski, K. A. (2018). Machine learning of brain gray matter differentiates sex in a large forensic sample. *Human Brain Mapping*, *40*(5), 1496-1506. https://doi.org/10.1002/hbm.24462.
[16] Soh, D. (2017, January 6). *Op-ed: The futility of gender-neutral parenting*. Los Angeles Times. https://www.latimes.com/opinion/op-ed/la-oe-soh-gender-neutral-parenting-20170106-story.html.
[17] Pasterski, V. L., & Geffner, M. E. (2005). Prenatal hormones and postnatal socialization by parents as determinants of male-typical toy play in girls with congenital adrenal hyperplasia. *Child Development*, *76*(1), 264-278. https://doi.org/10.1111/j.1467-8624.2005.00843.x.
[18] Stossel, J. (Director). (1997). Boys and Girls are Different: Men, Women, and the Sex Difference [TV series episode]. In *20/20*. ABC News.
[19] Haig, D. (2000). Of Sex and Gender. *Nature Genetics*, *25*(4), 373. https://doi.org/10.1038/78033.
[20] Harrington, E. (2016, June 1). *NYC defines gender as male, female, 'Or something else entirely'*. The Washington Free Beacon. https://freebeacon.com/issues/de-blasio-nyc-gender/.
[21] Goldman, R. (2014, February 3). *Here's a list of 58 gender options for Facebook users*. ABC News. https://abcnews.go.com/blogs/headlines/2014/02/heres-a-list-of-58-gender-options-for-facebook-users/.

Chapter 25

[1] Keenan, J. (2019, February 26). *Doctors: 14-Year-Old needs no parent consent for trans hormones*. The Federalist. https://thefederalist.com/2019/02/26/doctors-insist-canadian-14-year-old-needs-no-parent-consent-trans-hormone-injections/.
[2] Ford, Z. (2012, December 3). *APA revises manual: Being transgender is no longer a mental disorder*. ThinkProgress. https://thinkprogress.org/apa-revises-manual-being-transgender-is-no-longer-a-mental-disorder-8b0321f775d2/.
[3] Johnson, D., & Wagner, K. (2020, June 16). *Supreme Court Speaks: Title VII Forbids Workplace Discrimination Based on Sexual Orientation and Transgender Status*. American Bar Association. https://www.americanbar.org/groups/labor_law/publications/flash_archive/issue-june-2020/supreme-court-speaks/.
[4] Whitlock, J. (2021, October 7). *Gender Confirmation Surgery*. Verywell Health. https://www.verywellhealth.com/gender-confirmation-surgery-gcs-3157235.
[5] Levine, S. B., & Solomon, A. (2008). Meanings and political implications of "Psychopathology" in a gender identity clinic: A report of 10 cases. *Journal of Sex & Marital Therapy*, *35*(1), 40-57. https://doi.org/10.1080/00926230802525646.
[6] Dhejne, C., & Lichtenstein, P. (2011). Long-term follow-up of transsexual persons undergoing sex reassignment surgery: Cohort study in Sweden. *PLoS ONE*, *6*(2), e16885. https://doi.org/10.1371/journal.pone.0016885.
[7] À Campo, J., & Nijman, H. (2003). Psychiatric comorbidity of gender identity disorders: A survey among Dutch psychiatrists. *American Journal of Psychiatry*, *160*(7), 1332-1336. https://doi.org/10.1176/appi.ajp.160.7.1332.

---

[8] Mazaheri Meybodi, A., & Hajebi, A. (2014). Psychiatric Axis I comorbidities among patients with gender dysphoria. *Psychiatry Journal*, *2014*, 1-5. https://doi.org/10.1155/2014/971814.
[9] Budge, S. L., & Adelson, J. L. (2013). Anxiety and depression in transgender individuals: The roles of transition status, loss, social support, and coping. *Journal of Consulting and Clinical Psychology*, *81*(3), 545-557. https://doi.org/10.1037/a0031774.
[10] Mazaheri Meybodi, A., & Hajebi, A. (2014). Psychiatric Axis I comorbidities among patients with gender dysphoria. *Psychiatry Journal*, *2014*, 1-5. https://doi.org/10.1155/2014/971814.
[11] Ungar, L. (2015, August 16). *Transgender people face alarmingly high risk of suicide.* USA Today. https://www.usatoday.com/story/news/nation/2015/08/16/transgender-individuals-face-high-rates--suicide-attempts/31626633/.
[12] Dhejne, C., & Lichtenstein, P. (2011). Long-term follow-up of transsexual persons undergoing sex reassignment surgery: Cohort study in Sweden. *PLoS ONE*, *6*(2), e16885. https://doi.org/10.1371/journal.pone.0016885.
[13] Byne, W., & Bradley, S. J. (2012). Report of the American psychiatric association task force on treatment of gender identity disorder. *Archives of Sexual Behavior*, *41*(4), 759-796. https://doi.org/10.1007/s10508-012-9975-x.
[14] Batty, D. (2004, July 30). *Sex changes are not effective, say researchers.* The Guardian. https://www.theguardian.com/society/2004/jul/30/health.mentalhealth.
[15] Hyde, C. "Sex Reassignment Surgery for the Treatment of Gender Dysphoria", *Medical Technology Directory*, (2018, August 1), http://www.hayesinc.com/hayes/publications/medical-technology-directory/dir-sex707/.
[16] Centers for Medicare and Medicaid Services, "Decision Memo for Gender Dysphoria and Gender Reassignment Surgery", (August 30, 2016), https://www.cms.gov/medicare-coverage-database/details/nca-decision-memo.aspx?NCAId=282&bc=ACAAAAAAQAAA&.
[17] Person, E. (2008). Harry Benjamin: Creative Maverick. *Journal of Gay & Lesbian Mental Health*, *12*(3), 259-275. https://doi.org/10.1080/19359700802111619.
[18] Ubaldo, L., & Drescher, J. (2004). *Transgender Subjectivities: A Clinician's Guide.* WorldCat.org. https://www.worldcat.org/title/transgender-subjectivities-a-clinicians-guide/oclc/55106423.
[19] McHugh, P. (2016, May 13). Transgender Surgery Isn't the Solution A drastic physical change doesn't address underlying psycho-social troubles. *The Wall Street Journal.* https://www.wsj.com/articles/paul-mchugh-transgender-surgery-isnt-the-solution-1402615120.
[20] McHugh, P. R. (1995). Witches, multiple personalities, and other psychiatric artifacts. *Nature Medicine*, *1*(2), 110-114. doi:10.1038/nm0295-110.
[21] Ford, Z. (2016, October 18). *Johns Hopkins to resume gender-affirming surgeries after nearly 40 years.* ThinkProgress. https://thinkprogress.org/johns-hopkins-transgender-surgery-5c9c428184c1/.
[22] McHugh, P. (2016, May 13). Transgender Surgery Isn't the Solution A drastic physical change doesn't address underlying psycho-social troubles. *The Wall Street Journal.* https://www.wsj.com/articles/paul-mchugh-transgender-surgery-isnt-the-solution-1402615120.

[23] American Psychiatric Association: Diagnostic and Statistical Manual of Mental Disorders, Fifth Edition, Arlington, VA, American Psychiatric Association, 2013 (451-459). See page 455 re: rates of persistence of gender dysphoria.
[24] Cretella, M. (2016, March). *Gender Ideology Harms Children*. American College of Pediatricians. https://acpeds.org/assets/imported/9.14.17-Gender-Ideology-Harms-Children_updated-MC.pdf.
[25]Mozes, A. (2023, August 23). *U.S. gender-affirming surgeries nearly tripled in 3 years.* US News & World Report. https://www.usnews.com/news/health-news/articles/2023-08-23/u-s-gender-affirming-surgeries-nearly-tripled-in-3-years.
[26] Ellis Nut, A. (2018, February 28). *Transgender Surgeries on the Rise Says First Study of Its Kind.* The Washington Post. https://www.washingtonpost.com/news/to-your-health/wp/2018/02/28/transgender-surgeries-are-on-the-rise-says-first-study-of-its-kind/.
[27] Borreli, L. (2017, October 3). *Transgender Surgery: Regret Rates Highest in Male-to-Female Reassignment Operations.* Newsweek. https://www.newsweek.com/transgender-women-transgender-men-sex-change-sex-reassignment-surgery-676777.
[28] Lindeen, M. (Director). (2010). *Regretters (Angrarna).* [Two men in their 60's meet for the first time and discuss their respective sex changes, and subsequent reversals]. Atmo Media Network.
[29] Batty, D. (2004, July 30). *Mistaken identity.* the Guardian. https://www.theguardian.com/society/2004/jul/31/health.socialcare.
[30] Penner, M. (2007, April 26). *Old Mike, new Christine.* Los Angeles Times. https://www.latimes.com/archives/la-xpm-2007-apr-26-la-sp-oldmike26apr26-story.html.
[31] Rogers, J. (2009, November 29). *Mike Penner - L.A. Times sports writer - dies.* SFGate. https://www.sfgate.com/bayarea/article/mike-penner-l-a-times-sports-writer-dies-3209040.php.
[32] Morabito, S. (2014, November 18). *Trouble in Transtopia: Murmurs of sex change regret.* The Federalist. https://thefederalist.com/2014/11/11/trouble-in-transtopia-murmurs-of-sex-change-regret/.
[33] Wadler, J. (2007, February 1). *The Lady Regrets.* The New York Times. https://www.nytimes.com/2007/02/01/garden/01renee.html?pagewanted=all&_r=0.
[34] Russell, S. (2014, June 3). *Two-thirds of britons REGRET having cosmetic surgery.* Daily Mail. https://www.dailymail.co.uk/femail/article-2640543/Two-thirds-Britons-REGRET-having-cosmetic-surgery.html.
[35] Lombardo, F., & Toselli, L. (2013). Hormone and genetic study in male to female transsexual patients. *Journal of Endocrinological Investigation, 36*(8), 550-557. https://doi.org/10.3275/8813.
[36] Heyer, W. (2016, February 2). *50 years of sex changes, mental disorders, and too many suicides.* Public Disclosure: The Journal of the Witherspoon Institute. https://www.thepublicdiscourse.com/2016/02/16376/.
[37] Gayle, D. (2013, October 1). *Transsexual, 44, elects to die by euthanasia after botched sex-change operation turned him into a 'monster'.* Daily Mail. https://www.dailymail.co.uk/news/article-2440086/Belgian-transsexual-Nathan-Verhelst-44-elects-die-euthanasia-botched-sex-change-operation.html.
[38] Barber, N. (2018, March 16). *The gender reassignment controversy - When people opt for surgery, are they satisfied with the outcome?.* Psychology Today. https://www.psychologytoday.com/us/blog/the-human-beast/201803/the-gender-reassignment-controversy.

---

[39] Littman, L. (2018). Parent reports of adolescents and young adults perceived to show signs of a rapid onset of gender dysphoria. *PLOS ONE*, *13*(8), e0202330. https://doi.org/10.1371/journal.pone.0202330.

[40] Mikelionis, L. (2018, August 30). *Brown U. censors 'gender dysphoria' study, worried that findings might 'invalidate the perspectives' of transgender community*. Fox News. https://www.foxnews.com/us/brown-u-censors-gender-dysphoria-study-worried-that-findings-might-invalidate-the-perspectives-of-transgender-community.

[41] McHugh, P. (2016, May 13). Transgender Surgery Isn't the Solution A drastic physical change doesn't address underlying psycho-social troubles. *The Wall Street Journal*. https://www.wsj.com/articles/paul-mchugh-transgender-surgery-isnt-the-solution-1402615120.

Made in United States
North Haven, CT
07 March 2025

66540187R00166